# Breast Choices for the Best Chances: Your Breasts, Your Life, and How You Can Win the Battle!

## By Shawn Messonnier, D.V.M.

I0101937

## Acknowledgements

I am indebted to all of the health care professionals who were able to speak with me or provide research information for this book. In particular, I'm very thankful for all the help given to me by one of the naturopathic physicians at the Life Extension Foundation, Dr. Stephen Nemeroff.

I'm also thankful to my wife Sandy who encouraged me to share her story with all of you for her input on the book as well.

Thanks to my website designer Jim Klymus for his help in the technical preparation of the book.

Thanks to members of the Dog Writers Association of America for their input and help in choosing a title for this book.

Thanks to all those who work to find the best methods of diagnosing and treating and curing breast cancer.

Finally, thanks to all of you who fight breast cancer. Your inspiring stories and journeys were foremost in my mind as I wrote *Breast Choices for the Best Chances: Your Breasts, Your Life, and How You Can Win the Battle!*

## Dedication

This book is dedicated to my wife Sandy: May you continue to find peace and healing on your journey. You are one incredible lady. Thanks for making me a part of your life-I love you a lot!

To my daughter Erica: May you realize all of your dreams, keep Mom and me close, love God and thank Him for all you have, and never have to face the dreadful disease of cancer.

To the wonderful health care professionals who fight the war against cancer every day, especially those naturopaths who seek true healing and are always open to "something different" if it may help.

To all those women who have breast cancer and are fighting valiantly; to those who may have lost their earthly battles but won the ultimate eternal prize; and to those who may one day face this difficult disease.

And finally to 2 beautiful young women, Anna and Micaela, both friends of my daughter Erica, who valiantly fought but ultimately lost their earthly battles with their own cancers. May their families find peace and comfort in their loss, may those whose lives were touched by their courage find strength, and may they enjoy their rightful eternal reward where there is no pain or sorrow, only joy and love-we will meet again!

*"God is present in each moment and in each person."*

Daniel K. Lahart, SJ

The Chronicle of Strake Jesuit College Preparatory, Fall 2011

# Charity

There were 2 main reasons I wrote *Breast Choices for the Best Chances: Your Breasts, Your Life, and How You Can Win the Battle!*

First, I believe in women making choices regarding their own health care (for that matter, I believe EVERYONE should decide the best course of therapy for an illness.) While our doctors serve as a primary source of information, they should NEVER have the final say about OUR health care choices and decisions.

As a doctor, I readily admit I don't know everything! I don't have time to know everything, so I'm always thankful when my own patients provide me with research they have found that might positively influence the outcome of their diseases. I've done the hard research for you on the topic of breast cancer, and it is my hope that when properly used, the information in *Breast Choices for the Best Chances: Your Breasts, Your Life, and How You Can Win the Battle!* will save lives.

Second, I want to do something positive with this book above and beyond helping those who read the book. Therefore, I am donating a portion of the profits of *Breast Choices for the Best Chances: Your Breasts, Your Life, and How You Can Win the Battle!* to a variety of wonderful charities. Rather than single out one charity, I am going to use the profits to help those charities I find most in need of my financial support.
At least for now, 2 charities are near and dear to my heart. 1 Million for Anna is the charity started in honor of Anna Basso, my daughter's friend who lost her valiant struggle with Ewing's sarcoma. This charity will use funds from *Breast Choices for the Best Chances: Your Breasts, Your Life, and How You Can Win the Battle!* to help other young people also suffering from cancer.

Second, due to extreme financial hardships endured as their brave daughter Micaela, another friend of my daughter Erica, fought but ultimately lost her battle against leukemia, the initial portion of the profits from the sale of *Breast Choices for the Best Chances: Your Breast, Your Life, and How You Can Win the Battle!* will go to her foundation to help defray her family's extensive medical bills.

As an important part of revenue for these 2 wonderful charities comes from sales of this book, I simply ask you to encourage all of your friends and family members to purchase it. Doing so can save the life of a woman with breast cancer (and may help PREVENT breast cancer in a reader not currently afflicted with the disease) and save many lives through the good work of these charities and future charities that may also benefit from sales of *Breast Choices for the Best Chances: Your Breasts, Your Life, and How You Can Win the Battle!*

Disclaimer

The information presented in this book is for educational purposes only. It is not meant to serve as a replacement for consultation with a qualified healthcare provider. Therapies discussed in this book may or may not be beneficial for you or your particular type of cancer. Readers are responsible for discussing the treatments mentioned in this book with their healthcare providers before undertaking them.

Table of Contents

*"True progress in medicine has always, without exception, been violently resisted by medical authorities who cling to the beliefs of their times."*

Julian Whittaker, M.D., in the movie: <u>Burzynski, The Movie</u>

*"We tell our patients: don't make cancer your life. Move on with your life."*

Nicholas Gonzalez, M.D.

*"Cancer is a disease of the whole body…you've got to treat the whole body, not just the cancer…"*

Michael Galitzer, M.D., in *Knockout* by Suzanne Somers.

*"Every woman who has breast cancer needs to look at the conflict in her life."*

Stephen Sinatra, M.D., in *Knockout* by Suzanne Somers.

# Introduction

*"Dear Dr. Shawn: I recently lost a dear old friend to breast cancer. Kathy was told that the small nodes and lumps under her arms "were no big deal" because she was small-breasted, so she decided the military doctors knew what they were talking about and at first accepted their judgment call. But, as more nodes appeared, she decided to get pro-active and step outside military care and seek private care. But by then it was too late. Chemotherapy and radiation sapped her remaining strength. But before she died, she wrote a strong piece to women about the lack of concern the medical doctors place on breast cancer. It made me weep, but it also prompted many women in our town to get tested. She saved four lives and that is her legacy. Kathy was a native Alaskan and she was fiery, fierce and strong. I watched her wither away slowly and die tragically. Her last words to me were: "If only I had listened to the voice inside." Would it have saved her? I have no clue. I do know that both my older sisters are also breast cancer survivors and I feel I am sitting on a powder keg ready to explode at any time. It isn't a pleasant feeling.*

*I wish you luck with your book and I hope your book prompts millions of women to be pro-active and not trust the professionals- sometimes, they have no clue no matter how many awards hang on their walls."*

Sadly, this story is all too typical of those shared with me when it comes to the topic of cancer. While I believe most doctors care about their patients, they are usually overworked and underpaid and can make an incorrect diagnosis. In the worst case, the incorrect diagnosis costs a woman her life.

In our age of easy access to information, women (and men) MUST be proactive and take action. YOU are responsible for your health. You MUST "Listen to the voice inside!"

This book is NOT about "everything you want to know about cancer." There are many other books written about the specifics of various cancers and their treatments. Instead, this special book is about one woman's journey with breast cancer and one woman's journey facing a number of choices about the kind of care she wanted for herself.

As a holistic veterinarian who practices integrative medicine and treats numerous pets with cancer, and also as the author of one of the leading books on pet cancer, I was amazed at how much I still had to learn when my wife Sandy was told she had breast cancer. There was so much information for me to digest and absorb that it consumed a lot of my free time.

As Sandy has said many times to me and her friends and family members, if it were not for me doing the research and understanding the research on breast cancer, she is not sure how she would have known what to do regarding her treatment decisions. In all likelihood she would have followed the "standard of care," treatment recommended by her doctors for the "generic" woman with her type of breast cancer. In short, she would have been treated as "one of the crowd" rather than as a unique and individual woman with a specific type of cancer. Having someone there with her to ask the questions and find the answers was important to her, and is important to anyone dealing with cancer.

As a doctor, it's pretty easy for me to research topics such as breast cancer and understand all the nuances of the medical reports that I read. However it's not easy for the average person to do so. And when you consider that unfortunately conventional cancer doctors know very little about anything other than conventional therapies, it's imperative that you learn as much as you can about how YOU want to treat your cancer in your body.

Because you have more important things to do than spend a lot of time doing medical research, I've written this book to share with you the story of my wife's battle against cancer. With early stage breast cancer, Sandy had many options from which to choose and decisions to make regarding her treatment (just as you have as well.) In this book, I try to list as many of the different treatment options that are available to you as well as a number of suggestions regarding the therapies that she has chosen to take to assist you in your decisions.

Some chapters, such as the one on cancer surgery, are very brief since there is not a lot of information to be considered or options from which you can choose. Other chapters, including those on various pharmaceutical options and of course the chapter on nutritional supplements, are much more detailed by their very nature. Once again, this is information you are not likely to hear from your conventional doctors (but you should hear about them from your naturopathic cancer doctor, an important person who MUST be part of your treatment team.)

Keep in mind that YOU are an individual and YOUR cancer is very different from every other woman's cancer. You and your cancer are both unique and what worked for Sandy may or may not work for you. Information in this book is intended to provide education as well as a starting point for you to consider all of the many options you are now facing since your diagnosis of breast cancer. I'm not recommending you necessarily do any of the things my wife has chosen. I am recommending you keep your mind open and learn as much as you can to make an informed decision.

Keep in mind this book is simply a starting point for knowledge. Information can and does change, in some cases on a daily basis. Information in this book will be a guideline to serve as your introduction to the world of the numerous cancer treatment options you will face.

Regardless of where you are in your battle of breast cancer (maybe you were just diagnosed or you are several years past your diagnosis, or maybe you want to learn about ways to reduce your chances of developing breast cancer,) you can benefit from the information in this book. I believe that based upon my own experiences, as well as the research I have studied, that EVERY woman with breast cancer (or for that matter any person with any type of cancer) can benefit from being healthier due to proper diet, proper emotional state, and proper nutritional supplementation.

While much of the information in this book was discovered as a result my own research, I am truly indebted to other naturopathic doctors who have shared their experiences with me as well as lead me to research articles to support their treatment suggestions. I'm particularly indebted to Dr. Stephen Nemeroff of Life Extension Foundation (www.LEF.org) for his help and guidance in Sandy's care. Life Extension Foundation is a leading organization devoted to integrative healthcare and makes and provides a number of wonderful therapeutic supplements to help keep people healthy as well as assist in the treatment of diseases.

One final point: I don't want readers to think I am against conventional cancer treatments, as I am not. I use them daily in my veterinary practice.

However, in order for me to prescribe any cancer therapy I always ask the question, "Is this treatment likely to benefit this patient?" If the answer is "Yes," then of course I will prescribe that therapy. If the answer is "No," then I won't prescribe it. I ALWAYS talk with my clients to carefully explain all of the options, including the pros and cons, so that the pet owner can make an informed decision.

If conventional cancer therapy is something from which you think you will benefit, then by all means it should be a part of your treatment. If you believe the benefits of conventional cancer therapy do not justify its use (including side effects that may occur as a result of its use,) then it shouldn't be a part of your treatment.

I would enjoy hearing from you and your experiences with your battle against breast cancer. I wish you peace and love and the many blessings you deserve.


Shawn Messonnier, D.V.M.

# Chapter 1

# *What You Must Know About Cancer*

*"Breast cancer outcomes that matter most have not changed much over the last 20 years. The rate at which women are diagnosed with metastatic disease has remained constant for more than 40 years, and mortality from the disease has declined only slightly."*

National Breast Cancer Coalition's "Ending Breast Cancer: A Baseline Status Report"

October 2010 is the month our lives changed forever. My wife Sandy had been getting a mammogram done every two years. With no family history of cancer and with our concerns about unnecessary radiation, we felt that a mammogram every two years was adequate and would minimize unnecessary radiation to her breasts (mammography is a risk factor for breast cancer.)

I spoke to her during the day of her testing and asked her how things went with her mammogram (this was actually her second mammogram as her first mammogram, done a few weeks prior to this one, showed something "suspicious" but "inconclusive.") We were not worried as prior mammograms also had showed something suspicious while follow-ups failed to reveal any problems. I asked her how her mammogram went, and she said that things went well but that she would talk with me more when I got home. I immediately knew something was up since she did not give me a quick answer on the phone such as "everything is okay."

When I got home we went for our usual afternoon walk, a time for us to spend together, enjoying each other's company in a peaceful environment. On the walk, she told me that the doctor doing the mammogram suspected a tumor. A follow-up ultrasound of the breast area that showed "something suspicious" as well as a physical examination following the mammogram done that same day did in fact reveal a small tumor. Sandy's first reaction was that it was probably a small cyst or a benign lump, two things that are much more common than a malignancy. The doctor however, said that based upon her experience she was fairly certain it was actually a small cancerous tumor and that a biopsy would be necessary to confirm her suspicions.

A subsequent biopsy done in the doctor's office a few days later did reveal the diagnosis of "invasive carcinoma with a background of DCIS (ductal carcinoma in situ.)" At that moment our lives changed; we knew we needed to come up with a plan to declare war on her cancer.

The diagnosis was quite a shock to say the least. After all, Sandy had been very healthy, ate pretty well (minimal amounts of "junk food,") got plenty of exercise, had a good prayer life and a good marriage, and took several nutritional supplements. Of all of the family and friends we knew who did not have the "healthy" lifestyle we lived, we never expected that either she or I would ever be diagnosed with cancer!

Fortunately, because of my job as a naturopathic doctor who treats a lot of pets with cancer, we had talked about cancer in the past and always stated that if either of us ever got cancer, we would do two things: learn as much as we could about using an integrative approach to kill the cancer and keep our bodies healthy during and after our treatment, and visit with the doctors at the Cancer Treatment Centers of America for their input.

While Sandy's cancer diagnosis caught us totally off guard, there was some good news. Her cancer was caught early and she was given a great prognosis and is expected to make a full recovery (thankfully this is often the case with women whose breast cancer is caught early, and for whom this book is especially written.) The bad news of course is that she still was diagnosed with cancer and had to deal with that (and we will have to deal with it the rest of our lives.)

In this book, I'm going to share some of the issues we have had to face in dealing with her cancer. My goal is to educate all of you in case you ever have to deal with this horrible disease, and to show you the benefits of integrating diet, mind-body medicine, and nutritional supplements.

As a naturopathic/holistic veterinarian, I deal with cancer every day in my animal patients. Thankfully that knowledge has allowed us to tackle Sandy's cancer in a way that is unique and not commonly understood or undertaken by the general public. I'll be sharing what we are doing and what we have learned to provide you guidance if you or your family members are ever faced with a diagnosis of cancer, particularly breast cancer. While the main focus of this book is discussing the choices faced by women who are diagnosed with early stage breast cancer, the concepts and lessons are valuable for ANYONE fighting ANY type of cancer.


Chapter Lesson-Regarding cancer therapies, we really haven't made much progress in the war on cancer.


The cancer epidemic...

About 40 years ago, President Nixon declared war on cancer. His goal was to find a cure for this horrible disease. Sadly, we are no closer to reaching that goal today than we were 40 years ago. In most cases (a notable exception being some childhood leukemias,) we really haven't done a better job of treating or curing most cancers (obvious exceptions are small tumors that are removed very early in the course of the disease, in which case surgery alone can be curative.) While it is true that overall survival rates for people with most types of cancer have increased, this is mainly due to early diagnosis. People with (advanced) Stage 3 or Stage 4 metastatic cancer rarely survive despite the "war on cancer."

(The situation unfortunately is no better for our pets. While treatment protocols have changed over the last 40 years, most pets with advanced cancers are expected to only live 6 to 12 months following diagnosis, and that's ONLY if owners spend thousands of dollars treating the pet with surgery, radiation, and chemotherapy; in my experience adding integrative therapies usually allows pets to live longer than 6-12 months, often 12-24 months.)

The good news is that using an integrative approach changes these sobering facts and statistics. *Designing individualized treatment protocols for each person or pet with cancer, incorporating a proper diet, nutritional supplements, and other natural therapies offers a much better prognosis for the cancer patient.* We now have large volumes of research to show exactly how these natural therapies work in killing cancer and extending the lives of cancer patients.

In my own practice, the average pet with cancer, given a prognosis of 6 to 12 months of life expectancy from conventional veterinarians, typically lives 12 to 24 months or even longer. While never guaranteed, many pets with "incurable" cancers are cured from their cancers using an integrative approach to boost the pet's immune system, kill cancer cells, reduce the spread of cancer, and detoxify the patient.

The world of integrative oncology offers much hope for the cancer patient. Integrative doctors are helping people and pets with cancer live longer lives and in many cases curing cancers that are still considered incurable by conventional medicine.

It is my hope that by reading this book you will come to appreciate how important it is to diagnose cancer early and treat it properly using EVERY tool available at your disposal.

As I mentioned in the introduction to this book however, this is not something you should do on your own. It is imperative to find a naturopathic physician skilled in using integrative therapies to treat people with cancer to become a part of your healthcare team. There are numerous supplements that can help people with cancer but some of these may interfere with each other or with conventional therapies and can be inappropriate for use. The information presented in this book is to stimulate your interest in doing everything possible to help your battle against your cancer, and I'm not recommending any of it for you without the guidance and approval of your own naturopathic physician.

Breast Cancer Statistics (compiled from a number of sources including the American Cancer Society and the Komen foundation)

The average woman has a 12.5 percent lifetime risk of developing invasive breast cancer (US Statistics.)

The American Cancer Society estimates that over 200,000 new cases of invasive breast cancer will be diagnosed this year.

Over 40,000 women will die from breast cancer annually.

Breast cancer is the second leading cause of cancer death for US women (after lung cancer).

2.3 million American women have been diagnosed and are living with breast cancer, and an estimated 1 million have it but haven't been diagnosed yet (making early diagnosis critical.)

5-year survival is 100% for localized breast cancer (Stage 0 or 1) but drops to only 20% once it has spread to other organs (Stage 4).

70% of women who develop breast cancer have no identifiable risk factors.

Breast cancer is very common among American women; the chance of developing invasive breast cancer at some time in a woman's life is about 1 in 8 or 12.5%.

The American Cancer Society's most recent estimates for breast cancer in the United States are for 2011:

About 230,480 new cases of invasive breast cancer will be diagnosed in women.

About 57,650 new cases of ductal carcinoma in situ (DCIS) will be diagnosed (DCIS is non-invasive and is the earliest form of breast cancer, although many naturopathic doctors do not consider it as "cancer" per se; this is discussed in more depth in the Addendum on DCIS.)

About 39,520 women will die from breast cancer.

Death rates from breast cancer have been declining since about 1990, with larger decreases in women younger than 50. These decreases are believed to be the result of earlier detection through screening and increased awareness rather than more effective chemotherapies (while some doctors feel that the decrease in deaths may also be from improved treatment for early cancers, remember that there is no drug that can cure advanced breast cancer, and therapy for advanced breast cancer is only palliative to give the woman some extra (hopefully quality) time to spend with her family.)

Note:Sometimes deaths resulting from cancer are not recorded as deaths from cancer, which can skew the statistics to make it seem like fewer people are dying from cancer. For example, if a woman with breast cancer dies as a result of an infection she acquires during her chemotherapy, the death certificate may list the cause of death as "infection" rather than "cancer," even though it's obvious the infection was acquired as the result of her cancer. This is another way that statistics can fool you into thinking that the survival rates for various cancers are increasing.

Staging Breast Cancer

The stage given to the cancer describes the extent of the cancer in the body at the time of diagnosis and is based on various factors such as whether the cancer is invasive or non-invasive, the size of the tumor, how many lymph nodes are involved, and if it has spread to other parts of the body. **The stage of a cancer is one of the most important factors in determining prognosis and treatment options.**

Depending on the results of your physical exam and biopsy, your doctor may want you to have certain imaging tests such as a chest radiograph (X-ray,) mammograms of both breasts, bone scans, computed tomography (CT) scans, magnetic resonance imaging (MRI), and/or positron emission tomography (PET) scans (see below). Blood tests may also be done to evaluate your overall health and help find out if the cancer has spread to certain organs.

Since there are numerous other resources that discuss all of the stages of breast cancer, I'm not going to get into that here other than to mention the following points:

In staging breast cancer, your doctor will look at several factors including the size of the tumor, number of tumors, whether or not the tumor is in one or both breasts, whether or not there's any involvement of regional lymph nodes, whether or not the tumor has spread, whether or not the tumor is positive or negative for estrogen receptors/progesterone receptors/HER receptors, and most importantly, the actual genetics of YOUR tumor. Over the last few years, the growing field of cytogenetics has allowed doctors to actually look at the genes making up a woman's individual tumor. This information allows the doctor to determine the best course of therapy, whether or not chemotherapy is necessary, and the woman's prognosis.

In Sandy's case, her tumor was given a Stage 1 diagnosis, and her tumor was estrogen receptor positive (ER +,) progesterone receptor positive (PR +,) and HER negative      (HER -.) This meant she had a small tumor in one breast with no spread to other organs.

While in the operating room for her lumpectomy, the pathologist was able to do an initial microscopic analysis of the three regional (sentinel) lymph nodes removed with her tumor and did not see any cancer cells. However, further testing of these lymph nodes in the laboratory following surgery using immunohistochemical staining revealed micrometastasis (a small clump of cells) in her first lymph node.

This presented some debate over the best course of therapy. Technically, a tiny amount of cancer cells had left the tumor and "spread" to the lymph node closest to the tumor. However, her other lymph nodes were clear as were the various scans of her other body organs, especially the liver, lungs, and bones.

Here's the dilemma we faced: technically, Sandy's cancer had left her tumor and spread to one lymph node. However, the remaining lymph nodes were clear and only a small clump of cancer cells were found in the first lymph node. Unfortunately, there are no statistics to determine how to classify women in this set of circumstances. Cancer statistics look at whether or not the tumor is in 0 lymph nodes, 1-3 lymph nodes, or more than 3 lymph nodes (see more on this topic in Chapter 10.)

As Sandy and I and her doctors discussed, does it really make sense to treat a woman with a few cancer cells in only one out of three lymph nodes the same way you would treat a woman who has large amounts of cancer cells in all three lymph nodes?! Modern medicine does not have an answer for this which means it is up to the patient working with her doctor to make the best decision she feels is correct for her.

Note: Modern medicine does not have a lot of answers for many of the questions we asked. For example, we know there is tremendous benefit for cancer patients if they maintain normal body weight, eat well, get adequate amounts of sleep, enjoy life, and pray and relax. But HOW MUCH benefit is there? What is the difference in 10 year survival in women who share these traits versus women who are the exact opposite? No one knows, so it's tough to make accurate predictions about life expectancy following diagnosis when information is not available.

One of the things which aided our decision on how to classify Sandy (i.e., either as a woman whose cancer had not spread to the regional lymph nodes versus one whose cancer had spread to her lymph nodes) was the use of a genetic test called the Oncotype DX. This test (discussed further in Chapters 8 and 15,) useful for women with Stage 1 breast cancer, looks at a number of genes in **each woman's individual tumor** to determine the aggressiveness or lack of aggressiveness for that particular woman's cancer. Based on the results of these tests, a recurrence score of low, intermediate, or high is given. Based upon studies to date, women who have a low recurrence score and a relatively nonaggressive tumor will likely not benefit from nor need chemotherapy, as they have a very favorable prognosis without the need for chemotherapy. Women with a high recurrence score have more aggressive cancers; conventional doctors would argue that they would have a greater likelihood of benefiting from chemotherapy should this woman choose to undertake this form of therapy. Sandy's tumor grade gave her a low recurrence score which was encouraging and indicated chemotherapy was not necessary as part of her treatment.

Once again, while the results of the Oncotype DX test were encouraging, the interpretation of these results presented a bit of a dilemma. As of this writing, the results of the Oncotype DX test are only valid for women who have not had cancer cells spread to ANY regional lymph nodes. So in Sandy's case, we have asked the question again: should we consider her as a woman who did not have cancer that had spread to her lymph nodes (despite the fact that a small clump of cells were found in only one node) or should she be considered as a woman who had spread to her regional lymph nodes? In her case, we decided to consider her as a woman who did not have cancer that had spread to any regional lymph nodes in interpreting her Oncotype DX test.

Therefore, taking a look at all of the individual characteristics of Sandy's tumor, we were able to easily make the decision not to proceed with chemotherapy. Based upon individual tumor characteristics, we were also able to formulate a supplement plan for her which will be discussed in Chapter 13.

<u>Chapter Lesson</u>-Regarding cancer therapies, the best therapy for you is the one you feel is best for you based upon knowledge of your own tumor's genetics and individual characteristics.

*Sandy's Thoughts: It's truly amazing how many people are afflicted with cancer. I agree that it seems we're in a cancer epidemic and things don't seem to be improving. I believe all of us have greater chances of cancer due to our sedentary lifestyles, unnecessary stress, bad diets, and lack of nutritional supplementation. By focusing on health, my goal is that the information presented in this book will help you beat your cancer if you have already been diagnosed with cancer, and prevent cancer in those of you who have not yet had to face this horrible disease.*

# Chapter 2

## Understanding Cancer Treatment Statistics

*If you want to make God laugh, tell him your plans for your life.*

While it's important to understand breast cancer statistics, it's even more important to understand how statistics relate to treatment success or failure. Doing so will enable you to intelligently make a decision regarding treatment for your cancer.

For example, let's look at statistics regarding chemotherapy. In general terms, using chemotherapy to treat your cancer will reduce the chance of your cancer coming back or reduce the chance of you dying from your cancer by about 50%. Many women are surprised to find that chemotherapy does not guarantee a cure. However, if your oncologist is honest with you, he or she will tell you that the use of chemotherapy for any cancer treatment will not guarantee a cure but is designed to reduce your risk of cancer recurrence or cancer related death.

One question to ask is whether the reduction in recurrence of death by 50% is worth the treatment. That of course depends upon YOUR own statistics. For example, if your risk of cancer recurrence or death is 100%, then reducing that risk through the use of chemotherapy by 50% makes sense. If, however, the risk of your cancer recurring or causing death is only 6%, then a 50% reduction in risk only lowers your chance of recurrence or death to 3%. For most women, it would not be worth the expense and decreased quality of life that occurs during chemotherapy to lower their risk such an insignificant amount.

As you question your doctor regarding breast cancer statistics, remember that while there are general statistics for the "average woman," no female with breast cancer should ever be considered "average." Your goal should be to determine as best as possible YOUR risk of recurrence and death which will then allow you to determine whether or not treatment with a particular modality would be of benefit to you.

Here are several guides Sandy used in determining whether or not she wanted to use a particular therapy, specifically chemotherapy and tamoxifen, as part of her treatment regimen.

In general, the "average woman" with her type of cancer (without regards to the results of an individual woman's Oncotype DX recurrence score) has an 85% chance of surviving 10 years post diagnosis without a recurrence of cancer or death from the cancer following recommended treatment. Or to put it in negative terms, the "average woman" with her type of cancer has a 15% chance of not surviving 10 years post diagnosis. Note that this is once again for the "average woman." Sandy does not consider herself "average" and therefore wanted to try to determine **her specific risk** of cancer recurrence or death based upon whether or not she used a specific conventional medical therapy.

But for the sake of argument, let's just look at the statistics for the "average" woman with her stage of cancer for a moment longer. If Sandy used chemotherapy or tamoxifen therapy as part of her

18

treatment, it would increase her chances of living 10 years by 7.5% (a 50% improvement from the 15% death rate mentioned above in women who take chemotherapy or tamoxifen.) In her mind, it was not worth the decreased quality of life while on treatment nor the risk of serious side effects from either of these therapies to simply reduce the risk by 7.5%. Once again however, keep in mind these risk reduction rates are for the "average woman."

What about Sandy's potential risk reduction for either therapy? Using statistics based upon **her genetic testing of her tumor via the Oncotype type test**, her risk of death in 10 years following diagnosis is approximately 6% if she doesn't take chemotherapy or tamoxifen. This means that using chemotherapy or tamoxifen therapy would lower her 6% risk by 50% which would mean her potential real risk of death in 10 years following diagnosis is 3% (or put yet another way, using chemotherapy would lower her risk of death at 10 years by 50% AND using tamoxifen would lower her risk another 50%, so that her REAL risk of death in 10 years if she took both chemotherapy and tamoxifen is 1.5%). She didn't feel it was worth the potential risks of chemotherapy and tamoxifen therapy to lower her risk from 6% to 1.5%.

Keep in mind also that this risk is still for the "average woman" with a similar Oncotype recurrence score.

But what about women like Sandy who are on a good quality, mostly organic diet, exercise frequently, have minimal stress in their lives, have a loving and supportive family, a healthy and active prayer life, and are on numerous supplements designed to improve health and decrease the chance of cancer cell recurrence of growth? Unfortunately, while there are retrospective studies showing that women that do these things tend to have a better prognosis than women who do not do these things, there are no specific studies that can give us percentages. However, common sense would tell us that when patients do all of these things they are likely to have a decreased chance of cancer recurrence and death.

Putting all of these statistics together, it is likely that Sandy's risk of recurrence or death from cancer in 10 years following diagnosis without using chemotherapy or tamoxifen is somewhere around 5% on the high side and probably much lower due to her lifestyle and supplementation. Even if her real risk was as high as 10 or 15%, keep in mind that the "average woman" has a one in eight chance of developing breast cancer at some point in her lifetime (approximately a 13% chance of cancer.) Even though we now have to be extra vigilant and watch for a possible recurrence of Sandy's cancer since she's already had one bout of breast cancer, the chance of her cancer recurrence at some point in the future based upon her specific type of cancer and the genetics of her tumor, along with the numerous nutritional supplements and other positive things she is doing in her life to stay healthy, means that realistically her chance of dying of breast cancer is likely no higher than any woman who does not really have cancer, and likely much lower due to what she is doing!

While there are no guarantees, and Sandy knows there is always the chance of a future episode (that could prove fatal) with breast cancer, the odds are in her favor of living a long and healthy life free of breast cancer (and other cancers based upon her treatment protocol using her supplements.)

Finally, keep in mind that statistics can be easily skewed. For example, it's often stated that the 5 year survival rate for women with locally invasive cancer is 98%, but that includes women with early stage, minimally aggressive cancers that would have never died in 5 years from their cancers. It would be nice to find statistics that show how many women who were expected to die within 5 years from their very aggressive cancers are still alive following treatment. Since not all breast cancers are the same, while the 98% survival statistic is encouraging, it's misleading and doesn't adequately explain that for women with very aggressive or metastatic cancers, survival rates have unfortunately not decreased when treated only with conventional cancer therapies.

Of course if you have cancer it's a scary diagnosis and only you can decide which course of therapy is best for you. However, keep the following lesson in mind as you work towards a rational and hopefully non-emotional decision:

Chapter Lesson-Look beyond the percentage statistics to the real numbers and try to find statistics that are meaningful to you rather than the "average woman" to help determine your best course of therapy for YOUR cancer.

*Sandy's Thoughts: It seems like doctors are always trying to scare us with statistics. As Shawn points out, statistics given as percentages can be misleading. I believe the individual final number rather than the percentage is what's most important. Additionally, you must ask your doctor how to apply statistics to YOUR individual cancer. Statistics usually look at the general population rather than focusing on the individual, yet what's best for you can only be determined by focusing on you and your unique, individual characteristics.*

# Chapter 3

# *Why Did I Get Cancer?!*

*Two friends are talking. The first friend says, "I have cancer." Her friend then asks, "Is it serious?" The first friend replies, "IT'S CANCER!"*

*If it were not for the body's truly miraculous self-healing abilities, and the ceaseless self-correction process that occurs each and every moment within each and every cell, our bodies would perish within a matter of minutes. The mystery is not in how our body succumbs to cancer; rather the mystery is in how, after years and even decades of chemical exposure and nutrient deprivation our bodies prevail against cancer for so long.*

Dr. Joseph Mercola, Slash Your Breast Cancer Risk:Remove the Real Cause, www.mercola.com

When Sandy was first diagnosed with breast cancer in October 2010, to say that we were shocked by the diagnosis would be an understatement. After all, my wife is extremely healthy. She is rarely ill and rarely goes to the doctor for anything other than a basic checkup. She eats what we consider to be a healthy diet, constantly exercises, maintains a weight that is normal for her body composition (most cancer patients are overweight or obese, complicating their disease,) has a very healthy and positive prayer and spiritual life, and takes sevearl nutritional supplements each day designed to keep her healthy.

The first question she asked was "How can I have cancer since I'm so healthy?" Unfortunately there is no answer to that question, although we do believe that infertility treatments she had many years ago may have contributed to the growth of malignant cells in her breast. Additionally, knowing the link between emotions/stress and breast cancer in women (many women with breast cancer are described as having two traits: not establishing healthy boundaries with friends or family members and being women who over nurture others and failed to care for themselves,) we believe that a few specific stressful events in her life  (especially one that occurred at a time her breast cancer was forming but not yet diagnosed) also contributed greatly to her development of breast cancer.

All cells can become cancerous. Each cell has numerous mechanisms, via genes on the chromosomes in the cells, that affect whether or not the cell remains "normal" and noncancerous (via tumor suppressor genes) or becomes cancerous (via oncogenes [cancer genes.]) We are only now beginning to understand all of the different genes and mechanisms that cells use to remain normal or develop into cancer. As we understand more of cell biology and physiology, we can develop various therapies (drugs or supplements) that target the numerous mechanisms that allow cells to become cancerous. Due to the complex and numerous control mechanisms that allow cells to develop into cancer and spread throughout the body, it is essential to use numerous therapies to prevent these events from occurring (which is why multiple medical therapies or supplements are prescribed to help the cancer patient-one therapy only targets one or two cell mechanisms and the numerous therapies used by cancer patients target multiple cancer developing mechanisms.)

**Chronic inflammation (often called the silent killer since so many people are not aware of the amount of inflammation in their bodies) leads to numerous**

**chronic degenerative diseases including various cancers; genetics actually only contribute to a small portion of all of the diagnosed cancers.** Chronic inflammation is usually the result of poor diet and lack of proper nutritional supplementation. An easy way to determine your level of silent inflammation is to run a blood test that looks at levels of C-reactive protein (CRP.) CRP is produced in your liver and coronary arteries, then released into your blood when your body is fighting inflammation. Elevated levels of CRP indicate excess of inflammation in the body. Because most doctors do not routinely test for this (or other substances that can determine health or illness such as vitamin D,) it is important for you to ask that this test be done (see Chapter 15 for more information on special tests for the woman with breast cancer.)

Finally, another interesting theory on why cancer develops is the basis for pancreatic enzyme therapy perfected by Dr. Nicholas Gonzalez. He believes, based upon prior research by Dr. John Beard and Dr. William Donald Kelley, that immature stem cells develop into cancerous cells. These stem cells are difficult to kill using conventional means. Specific pancreatic enzymes (plus a diet tailored to the individual's needs and type of cancer, as well as numerous other supplements) help destroy the cell membrane of the cancerous stem cells, causing the cells to die.

Regardless of the specific reason that some of Sandy's normal breast cells became cancerous and were not eliminated by her immune system, physiologically the DNA in a few of her breast cells were damaged (cancer starts as DNA damage,) the DNA did not repair itself correctly (normal cells either repair damaged DNA or die,) the damaged cells failed to die (all cells except cancer cells eventually die, are killed, or "commit suicide," a process called apoptosis,) continued to grow (cancer cells utilize many unique ways to escape the immune system and the normal barriers in the body that usually inhibit the growth of cells,) and voila-cancer.

<u>Chapter Lesson</u>-Cancer does not discriminate

Cancer doesn't care if you are rich or poor, black or white, male or female, healthy or unhealthy. It is an equal opportunity disease and can strike anyone at any time. It is true that healthy people are less likely to develop cancer, and when they do develop cancer it is usually less likely to be a serious disease that is more easily treated. But the diagnosis of cancer reminded both Sandy and me that anyone can get cancer, anytime, any place.

Reducing Your Risk of Cancer

Several years ago I wrote a book entitled *The Natural Vet's Guide to Preventing and Treating Cancer in Dogs.* In that book, I suggested a number of ways in which pet owners could reduce and hopefully prevent cancer in pets (as is true with people, cancer rates are increasing at an alarming rate in pets, and many pets with cancer are now diagnosed at very young ages.) While there is no way to "guarantee" that you can totally prevent any type of cancer, there are many factors that can predispose you to developing breast cancer or have a "preventive" effect. Some of these such as diet and body weight are usually within your control; other factors such as age of first pregnancy or the number of children you have are not totally within your control. Still by having some knowledge of how you can increase or reduce your risk of developing breast cancer, you can become empowered to do everything within your control to try to reduce your risk of developing this horrible but yet oh so common disease.

Risk Factors for Developing Breast Cancer

Early age of the first full term pregnancy may lower breast cancer risk, possibly as a result of increased p53 suppressor gene levels or activity. The earlier you get pregnant the greater the protective effect.

Women who do not have children have as much as a 50% increased risk of developing breast cancer (due to longer periods of estrogen exposure and minimal progesterone exposure to the breast cells.)

Early menarche (first menstrual period) and late menopause are risk factors for increased incidence, likely due to increased total years of hormone (estrogen) exposure.

Women who use birth control pills have an increased risk of breast cancer due to additional exposure of the breast cells to estrogen.

Having suffered a miscarriage does not increase your risk of breast cancer.

Women with mutated BRCA1 and BRCA 2 have a higher incidence of breast cancer (mutations in the genes comprise about 5% of all diagnosed cases of breast cancer.)

Smoking increases the risk of cancers.

Increased body weight (obesity) increases the risk of breast cancer. Baseline obesity in breast cancer patients possessing the estrogen receptor–positive, HER2-negative disease subtype is associated with a 23% higher risk of recurrence and nearly a 50% increase in all-cause mortality. In fact, obese patients with this breast cancer subtype are at increased risk of recurrence, and once that occurs there's a higher rate of progression of disease and a shorter time period between recurrence and death.

Lifestyle stress increases the risk of breast cancer.

Alcohol consumption increases the risk of breast cancer (possibly by increasing circulating levels of estrogens or breast density): the more you drink the higher your risk. However, light alcohol consumption reported by breast cancer survivors in the United States was not associated with adverse outcomes in some studies (either additional breast cancer events or death). A moderate level of alcohol consumption, approximately one alcoholic drink per day, was associated with reduced all-cause mortality in the study, particularly among women who were not obese. It is felt that the quantity of alcohol consumed is more important than the relative frequency with which it is consumed. Because results of various studies have conflicted, it's probably best to limit alcohol consumption (especially sweeter sugary alcoholic drinks,) especially if you are overweight.

Poor diet predisposes you to many diseases as a result of inflammation. Americans have the highest levels of silent inflammation in the world, with over 75 percent of people afflicted. Poor diet can include: large amounts of red meat consumption and dairy consumption, especially since most meats and dairy contain estrogenic hormones and growth hormones which stimulate breast cells; diets high in sugar (Including high fructose corn syrup;) large amounts of fried foods; and diets high in trans fats/partially hydrogenated oils. Eating more (preferably organic) vegetables, fruits, and fresh (cold water) fish (such as salmon) is recommended. Organic meats (especially wild game such as bison, elk, and venison, and organic dairy products and eggs) are preferred in small amounts.

Women at higher risk of breast cancer include those who: have a known BRCA1 or BRCA2 gene mutation; have a first-degree relative (mother, father, brother, sister, or child) with a BRCA1 or BRCA2 gene mutation, and have not had genetic testing themselves, have a lifetime risk of breast cancer of about 20% to 25% or greater, according to risk assessment tools that are based mainly on a family history that includes both her mother's and father's side; had radiation therapy to the chest when they were between the ages of 10 and 30 years; have a genetic disease such as Li-Fraumeni syndrome, Cowden syndrome, or hereditary diffuse gastric cancer, or have a first-degree relative with one of these syndromes.

Women with a moderately increased risk include those who: have had breast cancer, ductal carcinoma in situ (DCIS), lobular carcinoma in situ (LCIS), atypical ductal hyperplasia (ADH), or atypical lobular hyperplasia (ALH); have extremely dense breasts or unevenly dense breasts when viewed by mammograms.

Lifestyle Stressors, Personality Types, Grief, and Anger

While there's no question that poor diet and environmental toxins increase our risk of cancer, many people overlook the effects of various stressors (including grief, anger, and unresolved personal issues, etc.) contribute to cancer. People living with internal and external stressors have changes in their neuroendocrine/hormonal systems, leading to increased levels of cortisol and inflammatory cytokines, which leads to chronic inflammation, a depressed immune system, and an increased risk of cancer.

Many experts, such as Dr. Douglas Brodie, M.D.,have studied personality traits of cancer patients and identified a number of common issues in many of these patients. These include:

Being highly conscientious, caring, dutiful, responsible, hard-working, and usually of above average intelligence; exhibiting a strong tendency toward carrying other people's burdens and toward taking on extra obligations, and often "worrying for others;" having a deep-seated need to make others happy and needing approval; lacking closeness with one or both parents, which sometimes, later in life, results in lack of closeness with spouse or others who would normally be close; harboring long-suppressed toxic emotions (anger, resentment and/or hostility;) reacting adversely to stress and becoming unable to cope adequately with such stress (Note:Many cancer patients experience an especially damaging event about 2 years before the onset of detectable cancer;) and having an inability to resolve deep-seated emotional problems and conflicts, usually beginning in childhood, often even being unaware of their presence.

In general, many cancer patients identify with the following emotions which can become "negative" if not dealt with promptly and properly: stress, anger, grief, and unforgiveness (holding on to past hurts and transgressions.)

For more information on this exciting topic of how personality affects cancer risks, I refer you to http://www.alternative-cancer-care.com/.


*Sandy's Thoughts: When I found out I had breast cancer I experienced several emotions: shock, frustration, and sadness. I couldn't believe I had developed cancer since I thought I was so healthy. Fortunately Shawn was there to provide support and do all the research that I couldn't do. I feel sad for women who don't have husbands like Shawn who is supportive and can understand the research behind breast cancer therapies to help guide their decisions. I know that women who read this book will learn a lot and be able to make more informed decisions, and that's why I really wanted Shawn to write it.*

*Even though my diet was better than most Americans who eat a diet high in inflammation-causing omega-6 fatty acids, there's no question that it could be improved. Additionally, it's impossible to escape from all the environmental toxins in our food supply, water supply, and air we breathe. However, I believe a bigger factor in my developing cancer were some unresolved emotional issues I had been dealing with for quite some time. Understanding this has allowed me to deal with certain issues and try to make myself "emotionally healthy" in order to prevent my cancer from returning or other problems from developing.*

*I also believe it's important to have someone like Shawn to be a health care advocate for you. You're probably going through a lot of emotions and are not able to speak up for yourself or make the best decisions, especially in the first few weeks following your diagnosis. Embrace your feelings, calm down, learn what you can, and do what's best for YOU! In most cases of early stage invasive breast cancer, you don't have to rush into anything. You have time to make intelligent decisions rather than emotional ones. Fear is danger, and fear causes you to make bad decisions.*

# Chapter 4

# Regular Checkups Allow Early Diagnosis-Mammography

*Despite the questionable effectiveness of mammography in reducing the death rate from cancer, regular screening is still recommended for most women.*

For most of the past two decades, the American Cancer Society has been recommending annual mammograms beginning at age 40. However, recently the U.S. Preventive Services Task Force, a government panel of doctors and scientists, concluded that such early and frequent screenings often lead to false alarms and unneeded biopsies, without substantially improving women's odds of survival, concluding that "the benefits are less and the harms are greater when screening starts in the 40s."

Most doctors still recommend preventive mammograms beginning for most women when they turn 40; women at higher risk are often recommended to begin mammography at an earlier age.  Women at high risk might include those who have a known BRCA1 or BRCA2 gene mutation; have a first-degree relative (mother, father, brother, sister, or child) with a BRCA1 or BRCA2 gene mutation, and have not had genetic testing themselves; have a lifetime risk of breast cancer of about 20% to 25% or greater, according to risk assessment tools that are based mainly on a family history that includes both her mother's and father's side; had radiation therapy to the chest when they were between the ages of 10 and 30 years for any type of medical problem; or have a genetic disease such as Li-Fraumeni syndrome, Cowden syndrome, or hereditary diffuse gastric cancer, or have a first-degree relative with one of these syndromes.

It is currently recommended that women at high risk of breast cancer (about 20% or greater lifetime risk based on a detailed family history or a history of radiation treatments at a young age), should get an MRI and a mammogram every year beginning at age 30. Women at moderately increased risk (15% to 20% lifetime risk) should talk with their doctors about the benefits and limitations of adding MRI screening to their yearly mammogram. Yearly MRI screening is not recommended for women whose lifetime risk of breast cancer is less than 15%. Due to the benefits of MRI testing, it may be that simply having the breast MRI done WITHOUT the mammogram is adequate (although most doctors have been so indoctrinated in the use of mammograms that you will need to be vocal enough to question the need for the mammogram and decline it if you feel that the MRI is all you want to have done as a screening test.)

However, keep in mind that while many breast cancers can be discovered through mammography (as was Sandy's cancer,) there are several drawbacks to frequent mammography.

First, for women with dense breast tissue, mammography often misses early cancers, allowing these early minimally aggressive cancers to grow and spread until they can be detected on mammography, often not until the next mammogram in 12 months or more. For women with dense breasts, breast ultrasound following mammography is critical in diagnosing smaller tumors or areas of DCIS (on Sandy's mammogram, a "suspicious area" was detected which was again noted a few weeks later on a follow-up mammogram. Ultimately, an ultrasound was needed to confirm that there really was a tumor in her dense breast tissue.)

Second, mammograms routinely detect non-existent tumors (false positive results,) meaning that many women undergo invasive biopsies needlessly since no tumors are actually present. If there are any unclear results on a mammogram, request a breast ultrasound or MRI before getting a biopsy. Mammograms also detect DCIS. Many women with DCIS do not need the aggressive therapies recommended for women with detectable tumors, even though many doctors often push aggressive treatment of what may be a premalignant (and sometimes benign) condition. This results in unnecessary treatment and expense.

Third, any time you receive a mammogram, you are exposing your healthy breast cells to radiation (with damage of the DNA occurring in at least some of these cells.) Radiation-induced DNA damage can actually lead to breast cancer, which makes many women wonder if annual mammograms are really needed. Due to radiation concerns and no family history of breast cancer, Sandy had mammograms every 2 years.

Finally, new research shows that for many women, especially younger women, the value of regular mammography is questionable. For women ages 40-49, the odds of dying from breast cancer over the next 10 years is 35 (35 women out of 10,000) if they don't get a mammogram but 30 if they do get a mammogram. For women ages 50-59, the odds of dying from breast cancer over the next 10 years is 53 (53 women out of 10,000) if they don't get a mammogram but 46 if they do get a mammogram. And for women ages 60-69, the odds of dying from breast cancer over the next 10 years is 83 (83 women out of 10,000) if they don't get a mammogram but 56 if they do get a mammogram. Approximately 500-2000 women out of 10,000 women who do get an annual mammogram regardless of their age will have an unnecessary biopsy based upon findings from the mammogram, and anywhere from 10-270 will have unnecessary treatment (chemotherapy, radiation, etc.) based upon these findings. These statistics make it clear that the decision for mammography, especially in younger women with no increased risk factors for breast cancer, is a personal one and should be decided by you after consulting with your doctor (who may push for mammography regardless of these statistics) and reviewing all relevant information.

There are several options for the woman who wants to minimize radiation-induced DNA damage from mammography. Note that I'm not specifically recommending any of these options as your circumstances are unique to you, but I do want you to be aware of them. Taking antioxidant supplements such as quercetin, curcurmin, and green tea a few days before, the day of, and a few days following mammography can reduce cancer-causing DNA damage. Having mammograms done less frequently (and starting as late in life as is practical for your situation) means less cumulative exposure of healthy breast cells to radiation. And finally, using thermography, which uses digital infrared imaging that analyzes body heat levels in and around the breasts as well as blood vessel circulation and metabolic changes that typically accompany the onset of tumorous growths, MAY be a viable option to mammography IF it is done and interpreted by qualified experts in thermography AND accompanied by a breast ultrasound examination (alternatively, a more expensive but sensitive test called a breast MRI can also be done in place of mammography.)

It's up to you to decide which regimen of breast imaging screening is best for you, and I can't make any recommendations other than offer you the information I've discussed. What I can say is that ANYTIME you have a mammogram (or any radiation testing or therapy,) you can minimize radiation-induced DNA damage using supplements including quercetin, curcumin, and green tea.

Chapter Lesson-Mammograms don't always detect breast cancer-request and get an ultrasound, especially if you have dense breasts.

Corollary-Mammograms expose you to radiation which will damage normal breast cells, which means mammograms may contribute to the development of cancer as well as diagnose cancer.

While "regular" mammograms may be important for women (and as I've mentioned exactly what the term "regular" means is open for debate,) it is much more difficult for mammograms to detect breast cancer in women with dense breast tissue. Sandy's cancer was actually detected by accident. She went for her mammograms and something looked "suspicious." A follow-up mammogram confirmed that the "suspicious" area was still present so the doctor wisely performed an ultrasound which easily revealed a small tumor in her breast. Were it not for her doctor acting on her suspicions and knowing that mammograms fail to detect breast cancer in many women, especially those with dense breasts, it is likely that Sandy's cancer would not have been caught at this early stage. While we were not thankful for the diagnosis of cancer, we were very thankful that it was caught early and will likely never cause a problem.

*Sandy's Thoughts: I do believe mammograms are important, but there is no clear-cut research to indicate what's the best age to start getting mammograms or how often you should get them. Additionally, women with dense breasts can have small tumors that are easy overlooked on a routine mammogram but could be picked up by an ultrasound, breast MRI, and possibly even thermography. I encourage women to talk with their doctors and work together to choose the screening program that's best for them. While insurance may not pay for a breast MRI, ultrasound, or thermogram (especially if they are not prescribed by the woman's doctor,) I believe you should get whichever tests are most affordable for you and which are most likely to reveal early cancer. Also, to reduce the chance of mammography causing cancer, I recommend supplementing with products such as quercetin, curcumin, and green tea a few days before, the day of, and several days following the mammogram.*

# Chapter 5

## *Regular Checkups Allow Early Detection--Breast Self-Examinations*

*YOU may detect cancer before anyone or any test does.*

In addition to receiving regular mammograms or something similar in order to allow early detection of breast cancer, regular breast self-examinations are also important.

I've always made sure to tell my wife to make sure she was doing regular self-examinations in order to detect any abnormal lumps. Unfortunately, she was not good at doing this. I asked her why she had not taken a more active role in "checking herself out," and she said that she really didn't know how to do a proper breast self-exam. In talking with her group of female friends, she discovered that NONE of these ladies do breast self-exams! Why not? No one was ever taught how to do them properly or what abnormal lumps feel like.

It's one thing to tell someone how to feel abnormal tissue (as doctors do,) but it is another thing for the person to actually be able to do that. Palpating (feeling) the breast for abnormal tissue is an art that can only be learned with practice (doctors spend a lot of time in school practicing palpation, learning to differentiate normal anatomy from abnormal anatomy, and regular practice is essential to be good at this skill.) While some gynecologists have life-like breast models in their offices that contain abnormal lumps which are very useful as teaching tools for women, many doctors do not have these models to teach their female patients (my wife says she was never taught by her gynecologist how to properly examine her breasts, even though she was encouraged by her to do so.) Additionally, the normal breast feels somewhat lumpy any way (more-so in certain women,) and many women have excessively lumpy breasts, making detection of small abnormal lumps difficult even for the most experienced doctor to palpate.

All this doesn't mean that women should forgo breast self-examinations; it does mean that gynecologists must do a better job, using life-like models of the breast, teaching women exactly what to feel for and what an abnormal lump feels like. Only then will women begin to understand the importance of doing regular breast self-examinations, which can mean the difference between life and death for some women with breast cancer.

Chapter Lesson-Most women don't do breast self-exams since they don't know how to do them properly. Gynecologists must teach women how to properly examine their breasts in order to allow early detection of breast cancer.

Current recommendations are that women in their 20s and 30s should have a clinical breast exam (CBE) as part of a periodic (regular) health exam by a health professional, preferably every 3 years. After age 40, women should have a breast exam by a health professional every year. It's also important that during this visit women discuss breast changes with their doctors, physician assistants, or nurses. They can also talk about the importance of early detection and factors in the woman's history that might make her more likely to have breast cancer. And of course, you should report any new breast symptoms to your health professional right away.

*Sandy's Thoughts: I know Shawn told me many times before my diagnosis of breast cancer that I should be doing monthly breast self-examinations. However, I never really knew what I was supposed to feel! While doctors tell you do breast self-examinations, it does require some skill and practice to know how to tell the difference between normal breast tissue and possible tumors. Have your doctor show you on yourself or a model how to do this. Had I known how to properly do a breast self-examination, it is likely I could have detected my tumor earlier. Since there had never been a history of breast cancer in my family, I never really took breast cancer screening seriously. Because you may pick up a tumor before your annual checkup, it's really important to learn how to do the breast self-examination properly.*

# Chapter 6

# *Understanding Your Surgical Decisions*

*Surgically removing the tumor is the most important conventional therapy as it may result in a complete cure and has virtually no side effects.*

For many women with breast cancer, there is good news:YOU get to decide which type of surgical procedure you want. Numerous studies have shown that for most women with early-stage breast cancer, a lumpectomy (removal of the tumor and a small amount of normal surrounding tissue) plus radiation therapy is as effective as mastectomy (removal of the entire breast.)

Note:It is standard therapy to follow lumpectomy with radiation to the affected breast, although it is possible that simply removing the lump without radiation may also be effective. It is my hope that more research will be done, particularly using the Oncotype DX test as a guide, to help answer this question as the test has helped provide evidence that chemotherapy and tamoxifen therapy are not always needed for women with early stage breast cancer following lumpectomy. At this time the decision on whether or not radiation therapy is necessary following lumpectomy is a decision that requires a careful discussion with your naturopathic physician (your radiation oncologist is obviously going to push hard for this therapy, whereas your naturopathic doctor does not have a bias.)

For women with a small tumor in one breast, your surgical choice is really more of a personal choice than a medical decision. In Sandy's case she wanted to preserve her breast so she chose lumpectomy plus radiation. In her case, recovery was quick and there were no postoperative complications or issues. With any kind of surgery there is always the issue of a postoperative scar. Time will usually make most scars disappear or at least become smaller and indistinct. Topical therapy with cold laser light or natural products such as Traumeel gel or ointment (or Vitamin E gel, aloe vera gel, or a corticosteroid cream) may also help.

Chapter Lesson-YOU can usually decide which type of surgery is best for you

NOTE: Some women are concerned about the possibility of breast cancer cells spreading as a result of surgery, and this is a real concern. Any amount of handling or trauma of the cancerous tumor, even something as simple as a biopsy to determine if the lump is cancerous prior to surgical removal, can release cancer cells.

To minimize the chance of cancer cell spread, Sandy began taking a supplement called modified citrus pectin (MCP.) Surgery increases the risk of metastasis by enhancing cancer cell adhesion if/when cells leave the tumor and spread throughout the body. Cancer cells that break away from the primary tumor utilize adhesion (sticking to other cells) to form metastases in distant organs. In order to cause harm or death, cancer cells must be able to clump together and form new tumors that can expand and grow (it is unlikely that a single cancer cell will form a metastatic tumor unless it attaches to the inner lining of a blood vessel or another cancer cell.) Cancer cells use adhesion molecules (especially galectin-3) to facilitate their ability to clump together. These molecules, present on the surfaces of cancer cells, allow cancer cells to adhere to each other as well as to latch onto the lining of blood vessels, which is an essential step for the process of metastasis. MCP may help fight certain cancers by binding with galectin-3 to help decrease cancer cell aggregation, adhesion, and metastasis. Taking MCP prior to, at the time of, and following surgery can help reduce the spread of cancer cells that consistently occurs when tumors are manipulated.

Sandy began her MCP a few days before surgery and continued it for several months following surgery.

Four weeks following surgery, she began her radiation therapy.


*Sandy's Thoughts: I decided to go with a lumpectomy versus a mastectomy for several reasons. First I really didn't want to lose my breast. While I'm not so attached to my breast that I would never have it removed if doing so would save my life, it is an important part of who I am and simply to cut it off because of a tiny cancerous lump made absolutely no sense to me. Additionally, the scar for my lumpectomy is almost invisible. If I had removed my entire breast and not had reconstruction done, the absence of my breast would be a constant reminder of my cancer. Since my cancer is technically cured and I don't think about it every day, I didn't want to have a constant reminder of it every time I looked in the mirror. There was some minimal postoperative discomfort following the lumpectomy but it's improving with time and with exercise. My advice for women is to find out where in your breast the tumor is located, where the scar will be if the tumor is removed, and how much of your breast will be cut. Then make your best decision on whether to remove the lump or remove your entire breast. My feeling is this: my breast is my breast, a part of my body, and I believe it's important to nurture your body. If it all possible, keep your body as whole as you can.*

Chapter 7

# *Understanding Your Radiation Therapy Decisions*

*Radiation can kill cancer, but it can also cause cancer.*

Depending upon your stage of breast cancer and which surgical decision you make, you may or may not need localized radiation therapy to the breast. For most women (especially those under the age of 70) who choose lumpectomy rather than mastectomy, radiation therapy is recommended by conventional doctors to kill any cancerous or precancerous cells that may remain behind.

While studies show that radiation therapy after lumpectomy significantly reduced the risk of the breast cancer coming back in the same breast, the studies also found that women with node-negative disease lived equally long lives after lumpectomy alone or lumpectomy plus radiation. Women with node-positive disease had an increase in survival if they had radiation therapy. The main benefit from radiation is to lower the risk that cancer might return in the breast, requiring more surgery and possibly other treatments.

For the most part, radiation therapy is no big deal for the patient. It takes a few minutes a day, five days a week, for five weeks, and then it's all over. In most cases there are no side effects. However, radiation can burn tissue, and a slight burning (similar to a sun burn) or chafing of the skin of the breast may occur. This can usually be prevented or treated by daily application of aloe vera gel, Traumeel gel or ointment, or something similar. This topical therapy must be washed off prior to the next radiation treatment but can then be applied immediately once the treatment session has ended.

While radiation therapy can be very effective postoperatively, it is not without potential harm. Radiation damages the DNA of all cells, not just cancerous cells. This means that a side effect of radiation therapy is actually more cancer in the future! In order to maximize the effectiveness of the radiation killing cancerous cells and doing minimal damage to the normal surrounding breast tissue (which can make radiation therapy safer and less likely to cause a secondary cancer,) supplementation with antioxidants including curcumin, green tea, and quercetin are very important.

Keep in mind that most conventional radiation doctors will NOT approve of your decision to use these antioxidant supplements during radiation therapy, and will likely try to strongly discourage you from using them. Their belief is that because radiation damages DNA in cancer cells by causing oxidation, the use of antioxidants during radiation therapy would make no sense and would potentially make your radiation therapy less effective since the antioxidants prevent oxidation.

However, large amounts of research have shown the exact opposite finding. **Using properly selected antioxidants such as the ones I've mentioned have been proven to improve the ability of radiation to kill MORE malignant cells while minimizing damage to surrounding normal cells.** While I never recommend withholding information from your doctor, be aware that if you choose to follow a naturopathic approach as I have outlined, your doctor may be totally opposed to this and refuse to treat you. The decision is ultimately yours. Based upon my own personal experience treating many veterinary patients, consultations with several naturopathic physicians, and a large amount of research substantiating the benefits of using properly selected antioxidants during radiation therapy, Sandy agreed with my advice (and the advice of her naturopathic doctors) and used the antioxidants we had prescribed before, during, and of course following radiation therapy. Wisely, she did not share this information with her radiation oncologist.

Chapter Lesson-Properly chosen antioxidants will maximize the ability of radiation to kill cancerous cells while decreasing the harm radiation therapy can do to normal cells. The decision on whether or not to take these antioxidants during radiation therapy to maximize cancer cell death and minimize damage to normal cells is ultimately yours.

*Sandy's Thoughts: I elected to do postoperative radiation more out of fear that I had and because my husband Shawn was also scared that the cancer could come back if I didn't do it, knowing that I was also choosing not to do chemotherapy. In hindsight, based upon what we've learned since my diagnosis, I probably would have elected not to do the radiation but simply do the lumpectomy. I'm not really sure how much benefit I got from burning my breast, especially since technically I no longer had breast cancer once the tumor was removed. Following radiation and surgery, my breast initially felt a little "weird" but this feeling is improving with time and it feels pretty normal now. Initially I didn't want Shawn to touch that breast during our lovemaking but now there is less discomfort if he touches it, although it still feels different from my other breast. The radiation was easy and I had no side effects other than slight redness of my breast and needing to take a nap in the afternoon. I was able to continue exercising which was important to me and I believe helped me heal from the surgery and radiation treatments faster. Because of the research*

*Shawn did, I took a number of supplements including antioxidants during my radiation therapy which we both felt would make the radiation more successful and cause fewer side effects. Because I knew my radiation specialist was a conventional doctor and not open to natural therapies, I didn't let him know that I was taking antioxidants.*

# Chapter 8

## *Understanding Your Chemotherapy Decisions:The Oncotype DX Test*

*"Current approaches to combat cancer rely primarily on the use of chemicals and radiation, which are themselves carcinogenic (cancer-causing) and may promote recurrences and the development of metastatic disease."*

(USA Department of Health and Human Services, page 56, patent #5605930, as reported in *Burzynski: The Movie.*)

*"History has shown that once a treatment regimen is in place and becomes standard, it can take a long time to remove it from practice, even when scientific evidence no longer supports its use."*

National Breast Cancer Coalition's "Ending Breast Cancer: A Baseline Status Report"

The diagnosis of any kind of cancer, especially breast cancer, is pretty scary. Immediately you start to question whether or not you're going to die and how much time you have left to live. Fortunately, with early-stage breast cancer, you do have some time to make decisions about your health care.

One of the decisions you will need to make is whether or not you will choose chemotherapy as part of your treatment. While many women, due to a fear of cancer, choose to follow whatever the doctor says and subject themselves to a number of chemotherapy drugs (all that have side effects including some serious ones such as additional cancer!) the reality is that some, if not many, women with breast cancer don't need chemotherapy.

According to some oncologists, *"Since chemotherapy is poison, why would we want to poison you for no reason?"*

Unfortunately, there is no way to predict 100% of the time which women would benefit from chemotherapy and which women do not need it. Fortunately, a new test called the Oncotype DX can make your decision easier (the test is discussed in more detail in Chapter 15.) This test looks at each woman's unique genetic tumor characteristics (the tumor is submitted for Oncotype testing following surgical removal.) Based upon the genetic markers of your tumor, the test does its best to predict whether or not you would receive substantial benefit from chemotherapy by assigning you a score of low recurrence, moderate recurrence, or high recurrence, based upon the likelihood that the cancer will return in the future. Women with a low recurrence score are unlikely to have a recurrence of cancer and unlikely to receive substantial benefit from chemotherapy. Women with a high recurrence score are likely to have a recurrence of cancer and likely to receive substantial benefit from chemotherapy. Women with a moderate recurrence score are unfortunately stuck in the middle and will need to make a decision based upon all of the factors of her tumor, including her recurrence score. In my wife's case, since her tumor type was considered less aggressive and she received a low recurrence score on her Oncotype DX test, the benefits of chemotherapy were not substantial enough for her to make the decision to take chemotherapy. Note that the recurrence score does NOT take into consideration the health of the woman or lifestyle factors (exercise, amount of stress, type of diet, supplements taken, etc.) that can influence future episodes of cancer.

The nice thing about this test is that it can save women from unnecessary chemotherapy. Unnecessary chemotherapy adds to the cost of treatment and has side effects including an increased risk of additional cancer in the future. While I'm in favor of using chemotherapy *when it's appropriate to do so and when the risks and expected benefits are clearly understood and accepted by the patient*, I often wonder how many patients die every year from toxic chemotherapy they got but didn't need. Some experts believe that as many as 25%, or more, of patients who undergo chemotherapy are killed by it.

The interesting thing about chemotherapy is that while it is designed to kill any cells that may have escaped the primary tumor site (the breast,) there is no guarantee that it will work or is needed. If there are no cancer cells remaining after surgical removal, then chemotherapy is totally worthless and potentially harmful. If there are cancer cells that have left the breast and spread to other sites in the body, there is no guarantee that chemotherapy will kill the cells as chemotherapy is not 100% effective.

In general, chemotherapy reduces the risk of cancer growing and spreading by 30 to 50%. In other words, if a woman's risk of future breast cancer (after the diagnosis of breast cancer) is 10%, then chemotherapy would lower her risk of future breast cancer to only 5 to 7% IF there are any remaining cancer cells in the body. In my wife's case, that small difference was not enough to convince her to ravage her body with unnecessary chemotherapy, a decision with which her oncologists concurred thanks to her low recurrence score on the Oncotype DX test.

In place of chemotherapy, Sandy decided to use a number of nutritional supplements that have been clinically proven to kill cancer cells. Her hope is that these supplements will be as effective if not more effective than using chemotherapy (which she does not need.) Because supplementation is safe and without side effects, the hope is that she will get all the benefits from their use without any negative effects.

*"The concept that "one size fits all" for all ER-positive breast cancer is clearly obsolete."*

Dr. Kathy Albain, Medscape Family Medicine

Chapter Lesson-Cancer therapy is very much an individual and personal decision. There is often not a "right" or "wrong" decision, and there are no guarantees or way to predict the future. Blindly following a doctor's advice is no guarantee of success. Instead, YOU must use all the tools and information at your disposal to make the choice that is RIGHT for YOU.

Chapter Lesson-Not everyone with breast cancer needs chemotherapy. Many women fall into a gray area where you will have to make a decision based on consultation with your oncologist. The Oncotype DX test can help make your decision easier.

Chapter Lesson-Most patients with node-negative disease who receive chemotherapy will not derive benefit, because they would not go on to have a recurrence even without such treatment.

Chapter Lesson-While there is good scientific evidence that adjuvant chemotherapy reduces recurrence and mortality for some women with early-stage breast cancer, doctors weigh multiple factors when considering whether or not to recommend adjuvant chemotherapy. However, many women do not need chemotherapy, will not benefit from it, and could die because of it. The path is not always clear and the decision is a personal one to be made after studying all of the facts and through meditation and prayer. As New York Yankee Yogi Berra once stated, "Although it is clear that a path must be chosen, it is unclear which path that should be." The decision is yours to make; make it with confidence and do what is best for you.

NOTE: The results of the Oncotype DX test can also guide your decision on the use of hormonal therapy with tamoxifen, as explained in the next chapter.

*Sandy's Thoughts: I knew that I really didn't want to have chemotherapy if there was any way to avoid it. I tend to try not to take medications unless absolutely necessary. Chemotherapy is poison: that's how it kills cancer. So if I didn't need to poison my body I wanted to avoid doing so unless it was clear that using chemo would definitely save my life. I've seen people get very sick and even die from using chemotherapy, so I really didn't want to take it. Fortunately the doctor who diagnosed my cancer, Dr. Miles at Solis, told me that it was unlikely my cancer would be a big deal or require chemo, which made me feel much better. My radiation doctor kept referring to my cancer as cancer with a "little c" (cancer) rather than a "big C" (CANCER.) As he explained, since my cancer was caught so early and since my genetic markers showed a less aggressive cancer, it was unlikely my treatment would need to be as aggressive as a woman whose cancer was more aggressive or had spread at the time of diagnosis. And when my Oncotype test came back with a low recurrence score, it confirmed my decision not to use chemo (and it also made my oncologist more comfortable with my decision.) After all, if there was no cancer we could detect in my body, chemotherapy would not be of any help and could harm or even kill me.*

*In talking with my doctors, and in reading the research Shawn did on chemotherapy and early stage breast cancer, it became obvious that many women with my kind of cancer will receive no benefit from chemotherapy and don't need it. Yet many women still get it out of fear. I know cancer can be scary, and I know some people with cancer need chemotherapy. But for women like me who don't need it, it makes no sense to take it. Remember that fear can be paralyzing and many people make bad decisions based upon fear. If you need chemo then take it (and use properly prescribed supplements to make the chemo more effective and reduce side effects,) but if you don't need it, I would encourage you to think twice before using it.*

# Chapter 9

# *Hormonal Therapy*

*National Breast Cancer Awareness Month was started by AstraZeneca, makers of the selective hormone-blocking drug tamoxifen!*

Following radiation therapy, it is common for premenopausal women with estrogen receptor positive tumors to begin therapy with tamoxifen (tamoxifen can be used for postmenopausal women but usually aromatase inhibitors are prescribed; women with estrogen receptor negative cancers do not need tamoxifen.) Tamoxifen is known as a selective estrogen receptor blocker (SERB.) This means that tamoxifen will selectively block estrogen from attaching to receptors on breast cells (but it also stimulates estrogen receptors in other parts of the body, as I will mention below.) By blocking estrogen's attachment to breast cells, the thinking is that normal breast cells will be less likely to develop into cancerous cells (as estrogen "turns on" the cells.)

Because of its ability to (partially) block estrogen receptors on breast cells, it is usually recommended that all premenopausal women who have been diagnosed with any stage of breast cancer that is ER + (estrogen receptor positive) take tamoxifen for 5 years to receive maximum benefit. Postmenopausal women produce small amounts of estrogen and would not benefit from tamoxifen or other estrogen blocking medications; women with ER – (estrogen receptor negative) tumors would also not benefit from these medications and may have a worse prognosis if they use them.

While studies have shown positive benefits for some (but not all) women taking tamoxifen, there are also potential problems with its use. Women taking tamoxifen for ANY length of time, but especially for longer than the currently recommended five years, have an increased incidence of two different types of uterine cancers (since tamoxifen stimulates rather than blocks estrogen receptors in the uterus,) stroke/heart attacks (due to increase coagulation of the blood which can predispose to blood clots,) a recurrence of breast cancer (usually a more aggressive type such as estrogen receptor negative cancers,) and the possibility of menopausal-like symptoms.

Comparing breast-cancer patients who received tamoxifen to those who did not, studies have found that while the drug was associated with a 60% reduction in estrogen receptor-positive second (recurrent) breast cancers ( the more common type, which is responsive to estrogen-blocking therapy) it also appeared to increase the risk of ER negative second cancers by 440%. This can be a serious problem since ER negative tumors have a poorer prognosis as they are more difficult to treat.

Keep in mind that as is true with chemotherapy, there are no guarantees with tamoxifen therapy either. In general, using tamoxifen reduces the chance of cancer recurrence or future new estrogen + breast cancers by about 50%. This means that if your chance of cancer recurrence is only 10%, using tamoxifen will (or rather "should" since there are no guarantees) reduce the chance to 5%. For some women, even this slight reduction in the possibility of future cancer is a good reason to use tamoxifen. For other women, including my wife Sandy, this slight possibility of a reduced future chance of cancer is not worth the potential risks that might occur as a result of tamoxifen therapy. Therefore, YOU will need to decide if the benefit of tamoxifen is worth the risk once you know the chances of YOUR cancer recurring (most women with small tumors diagnosed and treated as an early stage breast cancer patient with no evidence of the spread of the cancer are already "cured" and have very little risk of recurrence or new tumors, especially if they improve their lifestyles, diet, and start an aggressive supplement regimen; these women are unlikely to receive significant benefit of tamoxifen therapy but are susceptible to tamoxifen side effects!) Using the Oncotype DX test will give you a great idea of your possibility of future breast cancer. Keep in mind that about 90% of women diagnosed with early stage breast cancer will be alive 10 years from the time of diagnosis.

Here are the results of a study using the Oncotype DX test, to determine the benefits of tamoxifen therapy.

At 10 years following diagnosis, the risks for breast cancer death in ER-positive, lymph node negative, **tamoxifen-treated** patients were 2.8% for those with a low risk recurrence score, 10.7% for those with an intermediate risk recurrence score, and 15.5% for those with a high risk recurrence score.

 At 10 years following diagnosis, the risks for breast cancer death in ER-positive, lymph node negative patients **not treated with tamoxifen,** were 6.2% for those with a low risk recurrence score, 17.8% for those with an intermediate risk recurrence score, and 19.9% for those with a high risk recurrence score.

This particular study concluded that "in this large, population-based study of lymph node-negative patients not treated with chemotherapy, the Recurrence Score was strongly associated with risk of breast cancer death among ER-positive, tamoxifen-treated and -untreated patients."

As you can see from this study, women with a low recurrence score who took tamoxifen did in fact have a reduced risk of death from their breast cancer by slightly over 50%, but the ACTUAL reduction was slight (10 years following diagnosis, there were 97 out of 100 women who were alive as a result of tamoxifen therapy, whereas only 94 women who didn't take tamoxifen were alive.)

Of course other factors that contribute to a reduction in future cancer and death from breast cancer such as overall health and the intake of a good diet and supplements have never been tested in this manner but obviously favor positively in any disease outcome.

As a result of Sandy's low recurrence score on the Oncotype DX, dietary improvement (including flax seed usage, a natural phytoestrogen) and numerous dietary supplements including vitamin D, which directly kills cancer cells, and indole 3 carbinol (I3C,) which can provide a more favorable estrogen profile, Sandy has decided not to use tamoxifen as part of her therapy. This was not an easy decision and one we have constantly evaluated as I continue to research breast cancer, and was only arrived at after doing a lot of research on the pros and cons of tamoxifen therapy. Here's some of the additional research we found helpful in allowing her to arrive at her decision.

In one study, which included information on 80,273 women in 71 different trials of adjuvant tamoxifen therapy, the benefit of tamoxifen was found to be restricted to women with ER-positive or ER-unknown breast tumors. In these women, the 15-year absolute reductions in recurrence and mortality associated with 5 years of use were 12% and 9%, respectively. This means that for women using tamoxifen for 5 years (the current recommendation, as women taking the drug for longer than 5 years have been found to have a worse outcome than those using it for 5 years,) there is an absolute reduction in recurrence of breast cancer of 12% and a reduction in death of 9%.

Another trial showed that in women with ER-positive tumors taking tamoxifen, there was a longer time before the cancer returned but NO improvement in overall survival/mortality.

Several studies have shown no benefit or a worse prognosis in some women with ER-positive tumors who take tamoxifen. There are several reasons why this may be so:

When estrogen or tamoxifen binds to estrogen receptors in breast cells, the receptor actually changes its shape/conformation. Tamoxifen can lead to repression OR activation/stimulation of estrogen-dependent genes depending on the cellular context. Some tumors do not respond to or develop resistance to tamoxifen, possibly due to changes in uptake or metabolism of tamoxifen, loss of expression of estrogen receptors, expression of mutant or variant forms of estrogen receptors, loss of cofactors, modification of the estrogen response element, and ligand-independent estrogen receptor activation.

Additionally, a compound called cyclin D1 binds and activates the estrogen receptor in a ligand-independent manner and prevents its inhibition by tamoxifen. Breast cells in which there is an overexpression of cyclin D1 may also contribute to tamoxifen resistance. In fact, elevated levels of *cyclin D1* gene correlated with a 6.38-fold increase in relative risk of breast cancer recurrence and a 5.34-fold increase in relative risk of death following tamoxifen treatment (probably due to the fact that in the presence of tamoxifen, conformational changes occur in the estrogen receptor which promotes a stronger interaction of cyclin D1 with the receptor, possibly causing cell growth and potentially cancerous transformation of the cells.) Interestingly, elevated levels of cyclin D1 were found to be associated with a better outcome in several studies if tamoxifen is NOT used.

Other studies showed that strong staining of cyclin D1 in breast cancer cells is associated with inverse tumor grade, smaller tumor size, and improved relapse-free and overall survival of breast cancer patients. (For those of you who want to understand the science behind this, the beneficial effect of cyclin D1 correlates with its ability to repress the expression of the antiapoptotic transcription factor signal transducer and activator of transcription 3 (STAT3.) These results suggest that cyclin D1 overexpression induces opposite effects on breast cancer cell survival depending on whether tamoxifen is given or not. The authors of the study hypothesized that one possible explanation for this opposite effect of cyclin D1 may be that tamoxifen alters the interaction between cyclin D1/STAT3 and cyclin D1/ER: upon tamoxifen treatment, cyclin D1 can no longer inhibit STAT3 and that the resulting activation of STAT3 contributes to tamoxifen resistance.)

What is scary about these studies on cyclin D1 is that, as the authors conclude, because cyclin D1 overexpression is closely linked to estrogen receptor positivity in breast cancer, it is highly likely that premenopausal women with cyclin D1–positive tumors would receive tamoxifen therapy *even though clinical data has indicated the adverse effect of tamoxifen in this group of patients.*

Another study (A Review of the 1998 Overview Analysis of Randomized Adjuvant Tamoxifen Breast Cancer Trials, which presented results from the 1995 Overview study) came to the following conclusions:

"If the tumor has positive estrogen receptors, then adjuvant tamoxifen, for 5 years, should produce benefits, largely irrespective of age, menopausal status, nodal status, or prior adjuvant chemotherapy and is recommended. However, it was noted that these were proportional benefits, and the absolute amount of benefit would depend on the baseline risk of the patient, and might be relatively small in patients with small localized tumors of good histological grade."

In the studies, tamoxifen reduced all types of recurrence, but there was a trend suggesting that the best effect is against local recurrence (recurrence in the same breast in which the cancer was first diagnosed versus recurrence in the opposite breast or elsewhere in the body.) The overall risk reduction was 39% (tamoxifen reduced the risk of recurrence anywhere in the body by 39%.) Additionally, for estrogen receptor positive patients getting 5 years of tamoxifen, the estimate of proportional risk reduction is approximately 40% for relapse and 32% for mortality.

Finally, while many breast cells contain estrogen receptors of the alpha type, at least one study demonstrated that a high percentage (33%) of breast tumors express beta estrogen receptors. While there was no clinically relevant prognostic association of beta estrogen receptors, the lack of these receptors leads to a poorer response to tamoxifen. The presence of estrogen receptor beta (ERβ) in breast tumors confers a more favorable prognosis compared with tumors that contain only estrogen receptor alpha (ERα.) ERβ expression is usually seen in women who have not had spread of their cancer to regional lymph nodes, low-grade (less aggressive) tumors, and as a result usually show a greater disease-free survival rate. ERβ expression also showed a strong association with the presence of progesterone receptors and well-differentiated breast tumors. The presence of ERβ in >10% of cancer cells confers a better survival in women treated with tamoxifen. In conclusion, ERβ inhibits proliferation and tumor formation of breast cancer cells. For women seeking to "prevent" breast cancer (or "prevent" a recurrence of breast cancer,) food or supplements (such as flax seed or soy isoflavones-see the chapter on supplements to understand why Sandy is not taking soy and why it is not recommended by most naturopathic doctors) or synthetic ERβ-selective estrogens medications may be an alternative to selective ER modulators such as tamoxifen. Whereas estradiol binds equally to ERα and ERβ, phytoestrogens selectively bind to ERβ and recruit co-regulators to trigger transcriptional activation and repression, which can repress breast cell proliferation.

Unfortunately, it is not considered "state of the art cancer medicine" at this time to routinely stain women's breast tumors for estrogen receptor beta activity or cyclin D1 activity. While testing for these 2 factors would allow women to make a rational decision regarding the use and possible benefits/risks of tamoxifen, currently the "state of the art cancer medicine" is to prescribe tamoxifen to ALL premenopausal women who have estrogen receptor positive cancer, even though a subgroup of them will have a worse clinical outcome.

Because of the unknown status (cyclin D1 and estrogen receptor beta) of her tumor cells, because of her low risk of breast cancer recurrence EVEN WITH THE ADMINISTRATION OF TAMOXIFEN according to her low recurrence score on the Oncotype DX test, and the potential risks associated with tamoxifen administration for 5 years, Sandy decided not to use tamoxifen as part of her cancer therapy, preferring to rely on diet and nutritional supplements that may act as estrogen blockers and/or result in a more favorable estrogen biochemistry profile (this topic is explored further in the chapter on supplements.)


NOTE: Oncologists are beginning to recommend tamoxifen administration for ALL women that may be at increased risk for breast cancer EVEN THOUGH THEY ARE CANCER FREE, and some doctors are recommending tamoxifen usage by ALL WOMEN simply because they have breasts (since even having breasts puts women at risk for breast cancer.) Additionally, many doctors recommend tamoxifen (and surgery and radiation) for women with DCIS, even though many of these women may respond to natural therapies as many women with DCIS will not go on to develop invasive cancer and would be treated unnecessarily with conventional treatments (unfortunately, there is no way to know which women will develop cancer from DCIS and therefore a biopsy of the lesion is usually done to determine if the DCIS is more benign (which may not need conventional treatment) or more aggressive (which may require treatment to prevent the development of invasive carcinoma.))

While I am not claiming a conspiracy with the manufacturers of tamoxifen and similar medications, there is certainly a large amount of money to be made if every woman took tamoxifen for 5 years or longer! Based upon the science I have researched, I believe it's malpractice to recommend a drug with numerous serious side effects as a preventive, especially when MOST women will NEVER develop breast cancer and the proper diet and supplements may have a greater ability to prevent breast cancer than drugs such as tamoxifen.

Currently, our thinking is that Sandy may be able to get the positive benefits of tamoxifen therapy while reducing the risk of side effects through the use of nutritional supplements without taking tamoxifen, many of which also have estrogen blocking activity without the side effects that can occur with tamoxifen. Additionally, since her cancer is technically "cured" as her minimally aggressive tumor was removed at a very early stage (there are no tests to determine if a single cancer cell is somehow hiding out in her body waiting to grow into a new tumor,) the only potential benefits from tamoxifen therapy would be to prevent the growth of estrogen positive cancer while she is still premenopausal. We believe her diet and dietary supplements such as indole 3 carbinol and freshly ground flax seed will give her the same if not greater benefits than tamoxifen therapy without the side effects.


Chapter Lesson-If you choose to take tamoxifen to reduce your chance of developing recurrent breast cancer, it is critical to take supplements (such as melatonin and ground flax seeds, see the chapter on supplements for a greater discussion) to maximize the effectiveness of tamoxifen, while also reducing its side effects.


Chapter Lesson-Based on available research, it is likely that SOME women may benefit from tamoxifen whereas SOME women will receive no benefit and may be harmed. As is true with so many treatment options, the decision is up to you regarding usage of tamoxifen as part of your breast cancer therapy. As is true with chemotherapy, tamoxifen usage may reduce your risk of recurrence by up to 50%, but it's important to know your actual risk in order to better understand the maximum benefit from tamoxifen therapy.

*Sandy's Thoughts: As is true with chemotherapy, I resisted the idea of putting more drugs into my body. While it is true that tamoxifen may reduce the chances of getting a second estrogen receptor positive breast cancer, and using this drug may be the right choice for some women, there are also side effects of tamoxifen that sounded pretty scary to me, including uterine cancer and a second breast cancer that could be more aggressive and harder to treat (estrogen receptor negative) than first tumor. While these side effects are rare, I still did not want them to happen to me. Of course I could have chosen to have my ovaries and uterus removed; this option also made absolutely no sense. Why would I want to take out parts of my body just to lower my already low chances of developing a future breast cancer? Instead I chose a more natural approach to regulate my estrogen hormones. Hopefully through the supplements I'm taking that have actions similar to tamoxifen I will be able to reduce my levels of bad estrogen in my body and prevent a second estrogen receptor positive tumor. You must of course weigh the pros and cons of hormonal therapy for yourself and choose the therapy you think is best for you, but I prefer to address my cancer as naturally as possible through exercise, diet, supplements, and stress reduction rather than through more drugs.*

# Chapter10

# *The Little Lymph Node-What Is Its Importance?*

As part of the process of staging your breast cancer, doctors always want to know whether or not there are any cancerous cells in your regional (sentinel) lymph nodes. This is because doctors have always been taught that the presence or absence of cancer cells in your sentinel lymph nodes can directly influence your treatment and prognosis.

All doctors (and veterinarians) are taught in medical school that cancer that has spread to and is detected in the lymph nodes is not a good sign. We've all been taught that any time cancer is found in a regional lymph node it means that cancer has left the primary tumor site (in this case your breast,) has spread to the lymph node, and may have spread beyond the lymph node to the rest of the body. Historically, women with ANY amount of cancer in their regional lymph nodes were treated aggressively with chemotherapy and given a worse prognosis due to the likelihood that cancer had spread to the rest of the body. In other words, a "positive" lymph node (one in which cancer has been found) was a sign that cancer had likely spread to the rest of the woman's body, and she was treated (aggressively) with this understanding.

However, common sense plus clinical experience should cause us to question this assumption. Certainly a portion of women with breast cancer who also have cancerous cells detected in a regional lymph node have cancer that has spread beyond the node to the rest of their bodies.

But it is also likely that a portion of women with breast cancer who also have cancerous cells detected in a regional lymph node do NOT have cancer that has spread beyond the node to the rest of their bodies. In these women, the regional lymph node(s) has done its job, filtered out the few stray cancer cells that have left the breast tumor, and PREVENTED the cancer cells from spreading to the rest of the body. Unfortunately we don't have a test that can tell the difference between these two groups of women, but the good news is we now have additional information that can help guide your choices about therapy if you are a woman whose regional lymph node contains a few cancer cells.

While many doctors often assume that any cancer in a regional lymph node is a bad sign, fortunately, over the last 10 years or so, forward thinking doctors have begun questioning the significance of a "positive" lymph node, and their thinking is changing the way women with a "positive node" are treated.

As I've mentioned throughout this book, one of the dilemmas Sandy faced in trying to determine the best course of therapy had to do with her lymph node status. In order to understand her dilemma, it's important to have an understanding of how lymph nodes are examined after they are removed from your body and the significance of the findings discovered by the pathologist.

During a surgical procedure to remove a cancerous breast lump, several regional (sentinel) lymph nodes are removed along with the lump. These lymph nodes are examined by the pathologist at the time of the surgery before the surgery is completed. Tiny sections of each node are examined microscopically after being stained using a standard pathology H&E stain. In Sandy's case, all three of her sentinel lymph nodes (node #1, the lymph node closest to the tumor, as well as lymph nodes 2 and 3, the next closest lymph nodes to the tumor) were all read as "negative for cancer cells." This was the good news we were hoping for, and I told Sandy this wonderful information as soon as she woke up from surgery. The finding of 3 negative nodes meant there were no cancerous cells that had left her breast tumor and traveled to her regional lymph nodes, which meant it was unlikely she would need chemotherapy (and maybe not need tamoxifen therapy.)

As a follow-up to the screening of her nodes during the surgical procedure using the H&E stain, her lymph nodes were further examined in the laboratory using a more specialized staining called IHC (immunohistochemical.) This stain is much more sensitive than the standard H&E stain and can detect small amounts of tumor cells that might be missed by the H&E stain. It is fairly routine to do the follow-up staining even if the initial H&E staining is negative, just to make sure there is really no cancer in any of the nodes.

Following examination of lymph nodes stained with the IHC stained, they are reported as negative (no tumor cells seen,) isolated tumor cells detected (ITC, <0.2 mm of tumor cells seen,) micrometastasis detected (0.2-2.0 mm area of tumor cells seen,) or macrometastasis detected (>2.0 mm tumor cells seen.) In Sandy's case, despite not seeing any cancerous cells at the time of surgery using an H&E stain, follow-up with the more sensitive IHC stain showed micrometastasis (1.5mm) in her first sentinel lymph node (the other two lymph nodes further away from her tumor were negative for any cancer cells.) While this wasn't horrible news, it still caused us both extra unexpected anxiety as it presented a new dilemma for us regarding her therapy and prognosis.

So here's the dilemma Sandy faced: should she consider herself the same as a woman who had no cancer in her regional lymph nodes (negative) or should she consider herself the same as a woman who was found to be positive for cancer cells in her lymph nodes?

Unfortunately in cancer medicine, doctors base treatment and prognosis on whether or not cancer cells are found in the regional lymph nodes. For staging purposes, they group women as follows: no cancer found in any lymph nodes, (any amount of) cancer found in 1-3 lymph nodes, or cancer found in more than 3 lymph nodes. This obviously presents some problems as women with a few cancerous cells in one regional node are treated with the same aggressive chemotherapy and given the same prognosis as women who have large amounts of cancer in 2, 3, or more regional lymph nodes. Honestly, this doesn't make sense but that's the way medicine typically treats women with breast cancer.

So the dilemma/question Sandy faced was this: what is the significance of having just a few cancer cells (micrometastasis) in only one lymph node, which happened to be the lymph node closest to her actual cancerous tumor? If the other 2 nodes were free of cancer, wouldn't this be encouraging since cancer cells were only found in small amounts in the node closest to the tumor? Is it possible that only a few cells were found in the first lymph node and actually trapped by the lymph node, preventing any cancer from leaving her nodes and travelling to the rest of her body? If this was the case, additional chemotherapy and/or tamoxifen therapy would probably not be necessary, would be overkill, and might actually cause side effects (including a greater chance of MORE cancer in the future!)

At the time of Sandy's diagnosis, no one had the answer to the significance of microscopic amounts of cancer cells appearing in one or two sentinel lymph nodes. There was ongoing research to try to determine the significance of this finding, but the results had not yet been published.

Now, however, groundbreaking research can provide women data to help them determine their best course of treatment if small amounts of cancer cells are found in a sentinel lymph node.

As reported in the New England Journal of Medicine (online 19 Jan 2011,) Dr. Donald L. Weaver started this research about 10 years ago in an attempt to answer the following questions:

How many women, whose lymph nodes are determined to be negative for cancer based upon routine H&E staining, actually have cancer cells in their sentinel lymph nodes that might be detected with the more sensitive IHC staining?

What is the significance of finding small number of tumor cells in the sentinel lymph nodes if they are only found with IHC staining but not with the more commonly and routinely performed H&E staining?

Should IHC staining be done routinely, adding to the cost of cancer diagnosis, and what is the benefit of doing it or what is the risk of not doing it?

In this groundbreaking study, Dr. Weaver studied almost 4000 women over a ten-year period of time. In order to be included in the study, these women had to have early-stage breast cancer with negative lymph nodes based upon H&E staining. He then did the more sensitive IHC staining on their sentinel lymph nodes without revealing the results to their oncologists. The oncologists prescribed treatments without knowing the results of the IHC staining, instead only basing treatment upon negative findings from the routine H&E staining (and the specific characteristics of each woman's tumor.) In this study, most of the women were treated following surgery with radiation and chemotherapy or tamoxifen therapy (usually based upon their tumor's individual characteristics, including their recurrence scores from the Oncotype DX test.)

The goal of this study was to determine survival at 5 years following diagnosis, and take a look at whether there is a difference in survival in women whose negative lymph node diagnosis based upon H&E staining would change if their IHC staining was positive or negative.

The results of the study will prove surprising for many oncologists who believe that the presence of any amount of cancer in the sentinel lymph nodes automatically worsens a woman's prognosis and indicates that a more aggressive form of treatment be used.

In the 3,887 participants who were enrolled in Dr. Weaver's study, the results showed that occult metastases (cancer cells only found when using the IHC staining but not found when using the H&E staining) were found in 15.9% of patients whose initial sentinel node biopsy tested negative for cancer. This means that approximately 84% of women whose lymph nodes are determined to be "negative for cancer" in the operating room remain negative when using the more sensitive IHC staining. Even more dramatic however was the five-year survival rate among women who initially tested negative for cancer using the H&E stain but were found to be positive based upon IHC stain. Here are the actual findings from the study:

At 5 years following diagnosis, among patients with occult metastases, 94.6% were alive, 86.4% were free of recurrence (local, regional, or metastatic disease), and 89.7% had not developed metastatic disease. For patients without detectable occult metastases the results were 95.8%, 89.2%, and 92.5%, respectively.

The researchers concluded that:

The data did not indicate a clinical benefit of immunohistochemical analysis of initially negative sentinel nodes in patients with early stage breast cancer. While there is nothing wrong with using IHC staining as a follow-up test (other than the increased cost of the test,) the findings of a positive lymph node on IHC testing that was negative on H&E testing should be interpreted with caution and may cause undue anxiety for women with small amounts of cancer cells in an isolated sentinel lymph node.

Pathologists shouldn't continue to look for micrometastases when the initial evaluation is negative and oncologists shouldn't treat patients any differently or change therapy exclusively based on micrometastases.

Micrometastases are so small that they have very little impact on outcome - only 1.2% at five years.

Micrometastasis doesn't substantially increase the risk of cancer recurrence or decrease overall survival in breast cancer patients whose sentinel nodes were initially negative for cancer based upon H&E staining in the surgery room.

And the good news is that this groundbreaking study is backed up by findings from another one. A recent analysis of data from the National Cancer Institute's Surveillance, Epidemiology, and End Results (SEER) national cancer database has demonstrated that the presence of micrometastases no larger than 2.0 mm in lymph nodes is associated with an overall decrease in survival at 10 years of only 1% for tumors no larger than 2 cm (T1,) 6% for tumors larger than 2 cm but smaller than 5 cm (T2,), and 2% for tumors larger than 5 cm (T3,) compared to patients with no nodal metastases. Interestingly, a large retrospective analysis of data from California and Massachusetts demonstrated no impact on 15-year mortality estimates in any tumor size category when only a single lymph node contained any size metastasis.

One word of caution: Dr. Weaver, in his study, did mention that "multivariate analysis suggests that multiple factors (e.g., age and tumor size) influence the prevalence of occult metastases and the outcome, and that local radiation therapy and adjuvant systemic therapy, particularly endocrine therapy, attenuate the unfavorable effect of occult metastases." For women treated with chemotherapy and/or tamoxifen therapy, the presence of ITC's or micrometastasis did not influence outcome. For women treated without chemotherapy or tamoxifen, results were not available, although overall the study showed no real negative effects when women were treated by their oncologists based upon tumor characteristics (such as using the results of the Oncotype DX test and hormone receptor status of the tumor) under the presumption that their lymph nodes were negative.

Chapter Lesson-All of these studies have come to the same conclusion: the primary tumor characteristics are MORE important than whether or not there is involvement of the sentinel lymph nodes when minimal nodal tumor burden is present, especially when standard therapies are used based upon the tumor's specific characteristics. Ultimately it is still up to each woman to decide if chemotherapy and/or tamoxifen therapy might be helpful or harmful based upon her individual tumor's characteristics without giving too much significance to small amounts of cancer cells in 1 regional lymph node.

*Sandy's Thoughts:The first thing I wanted to know when I woke up from surgery was whether or not there was any cancer in my lymph nodes. Based upon what the doctors had told me prior to surgery, I was pretty sure the nodes would be clean but really needed to hear it from Shawn. When I woke up I asked him if the nodes were clean and he said yes. I was really happy and able to finally relax for the first time following my diagnosis.*

*Unfortunately, the good news was to only last for a few days. After Shawn got off the phone with the surgeon a few days into my postoperative recovery, he told me that they had detected a few cancer cells in the first sentinel lymph node using special staining procedures. I wasn't happy to hear this, and it did create fear and uncertainty. What did it mean? Was I now going to need chemotherapy? Would it affect my prognosis? All of the questions I thought had been answered following surgery were now resurfacing. It also meant that Shawn would need to do more research to help me understand what this new finding meant. We both found out that the finding of a few cancer cells in a single lymph node presented a medical dilemma: doctors really didn't know what it meant or how to properly advise women on their treatment. Should I be considered and treated like women with negative lymph nodes since all of my other nodes were clear, and there were only microscopic amounts of cancer in the first lymph node (and these could only be seen with a special stain?) Or should I be treated the same as women with large amounts of cancer in all of their lymph nodes (as some doctors choose to do?) This uncertainty caused a certain amount of anxiety for me. I chose to stay positive and consider myself as node negative and as having a good prognosis based upon my tumor characteristics and Oncotype score. As Shawn did more research he discovered that while this topic is still controversial with no clear-cut answers, there were some encouraging findings as he mentioned above. While I don't know what the future holds, I do believe that the finding of small amounts of cancer cells in only 1 lymph node will prove not to be a big deal for me.*

# Chapter 11

# *Understanding the Importance of Nutrition*

*"Let food be your medicine."* Hippocrates

Regardless of the kind of care chosen by the cancer patient, a proper cancer-fighting diet is the foundation upon which other treatments are built.

Fortunately for Sandy, her diet was already better than 99% of Americans at the time of her diagnosis. She eats mainly fresh food (organic when possible, which minimizes her exposure to pesticides/antibiotics/estrogens/growth hormone that are often used in the commercial production of meats, vegetables, and fruits) minimizes her sugar intake (and avoids toxic sugar substitutes such as high fructose corn syrup,) and eats only minimal amounts of packaged food (always reading the labels to avoid, when possible, the addition of harmful inflammatory-producing ingredients such as high fructose corn syrup and partially hydrogenated vegetable oils.)

The best diet for cancer patients relies on whole grains with a low glycemic index (high insulin levels, associated with ingestion of foods with a high glycemic index, produce inflammation and can lead to cancer formation, so minimizing refined high glycemic starches and carbohydrates is important.) Fresh vegetables, especially cruciferous vegetables such as broccoli, cauliflower, brussel sprouts, and kale are loaded with antioxidants and cancer fighting chemicals such as indole 3 carbinol (I3C.) Dark-colored fruits (berries) are also full of phytonutrients that reduce inflammation and oxidation and help fight cancer. Red meat (especially hormone and antibiotic-loaded/grain-fed beef) has been linked to the promotion of cancer and other inflammatory diseases, so Sandy (who was never a big red meat eater anyway) is limiting her consumption of red meat (usually naturally raised and/or organic, grass-fed beef, bison, poultry, and wild game) to ideally no more than one meal per day. Our favorite source for this kind of meat is Blackwing Meats (http://www.blackwing.com/index.php)

(An alternative look at diet is part of the protocol developed by Dr. Nicholas Gonzalez. He has found that certain people, and certain cancers, respond better with a greater proportion of vegetables and fruits in their diets whereas other people and cancers respond better with a greater proportion of red meat in their diets. This is done to help the patient develop the proper pH in the body, which is important to help kill cancer cells. And since every patient and every cancer is different, it's important to put the right fuel in the right body, based upon testing done by Dr. Gonzalez. However, unless you are being treated by Dr. Gonzalez and have a diet specifically prescribed for you, it is better to reduce the amount of red meat in your diet and increase the amounts of vegetables and fruits in your diet unless otherwise instructed by your naturopathic physician.)

Many meats, especially beef (that is not raised organically) is injected with estrogens to accelerate growth and add fat to the steer. Obviously women with breast cancer should not eat commercially raised beef as they need to limit their exposure to exogenous estrogens.

Commercially raised (not organically raised) dairy cattle are usually injected with genetically engineered growth hormone (rBGH.) This hormone causes the dairy cattle to increase the amount of milk they produce. While allowed in dairy cattle in the US, it is banned in many countries due to its danger to human health. In addition to causing problems in cattle injected with growth hormone (such as mastitis,) it causes increased levels of insulin growth factor-1 (IGF-1) in people, which can contribute to cancer. For example, the 1998 Harvard Nurse Health Study showed that premenopausal women with elevated IGF-1 levels had up to a seven-fold increase in breast cancer, and women younger than 35 years of age who have elevated levels of IGF-1 and develop breast cancer tend to develop more aggressive forms of breast cancer.

IGF-1 blocks your body's natural defense mechanisms against early microscopic cancers by preventing apoptosis (death) of cancer cells. While Sandy rarely drinks milk (she does use some on her cereal in the morning, combining it with coconut milk,) she does occasionally eat yogurt and cheese (and very rarely ice cream.) As much as possible, we try to purchase organic dairy products to limit our exposure to milk from cattle treated with rBGH.

Note:Many commercial dairy products specifically say on their labels that there is no difference in dairy cattle treated with rBGH and those not treated, but don't believe it.

Fish, especially cold water fish high in omega-3 fatty acids such as salmon, sardines, herring, anchovies, tuna, and sablefish, are also an important part of the cancer patient's diet (see more about the benefit of fish oil in the chapter on supplements.)

Wild salmon is so much better for you than farmed salmon, and as far as wild salmon goes, your best bet is wild caught Pacific salmon from Alaska (such as sockeye, king/chinook, silver/coho, pink.) In terms of sustainability, availability, and purity, wild Atlantic salmon is an endangered and/or threatened species, and is virtually unavailable in stores.

There are several reasons to choose wild salmon and avoid farmed salmon: salmon farming has damaged or eliminated wild salmon wherever it is practiced, by spreading disease; farm-raised salmon (usually Atlantic salmon) is raised with veterinary drugs including pesticides and antibiotics; although farmed salmon has about as much omega-3 fat as wild salmon, farmed salmon's grain/soy-based food give it unnaturally high levels of omega-6 fatty acids, which are pro-inflammatory and compete with omega-3s for absorption; farmed salmon gets its orange hue from synthetic versions of canthaxanthin (used in tanning pills) and astaxanthin (the carotene-class antioxidants that wild salmon get from the crustaceans in their diets;) compared with natural astaxanthin (found in wild salmon,) synthetic astaxanthin behaves differently in the human body and may not provide the same health benefits; farmed salmon can contain levels of canthaxanthin high enough to expose some consumers to amounts in excess of the European Union's Acceptable Daily Intake; and consumed in excess, canthaxanthin can lead to an eye disorder called canthaxanthin retinopathy, and has also been reported to cause liver injury and a severe itching condition called urticarial (wild Pacific salmon contain lots of astaxanthin, but very little canthaxanthin.)

We wanted the best, freshest wild salmon we could find. Fortunately, a company called Vital Choice (http://www.vitalchoice.com) sells the best freshly caught wild salmon from the waters of Alaska. They freeze it within hours of catching it and ship it on dry ice to your home. It is simply the best salmon we've ever eaten, regardless of whether we are eating their smoked salmon, fresh salmon portions, or wonderful salmon burger. We try to eat at least one meal a week with this salmon, cooking it a variety of ways and adding it to a fresh leafy green salad topped with homemade virgin olive oil and balsamic vinegar dressing. We also like the Vital Choice smoked salmon with our breakfast in the morning or at lunch mixed with organic greens to make a great salad.

Finally, one of the most important changes to Sandy's diet was the addition of freshly ground flaxseed. While she was already adding some flaxseed to her daily diet at the time of her cancer diagnosis, the amount was lower than needed to help fight her breast cancer. Studies have shown that 3 to 4 tablespoons of **freshly ground** brown (or golden) flaxseed per day can effectively kill breast cancer cells (by inhibiting human breast cancer growth and metastasis and down-regulating the expression of insulin-like growth factor and epidermal growth factor receptor.) It's important to freshly grind the flaxseed as the omega-3 oils degrade within a few days of grinding. Freshly ground flaxseed should be kept refrigerated to slow down the degradation of the natural oils in the flaxseed (see the chapter on supplements for more about the health benefits of flax seed.)

Because Sandy's diet was already good at the time of her diagnosis, it's been very easy for us to make the few changes necessary to supercharge her diet (eating out poses challenges, as does eating at the homes of friends; however, since our diet is pretty good when we are eating at home, we don't worry too much about eating out or when friends are hosting a get-together.)

Sadly, most people in our country eat a pro-inflammatory diet that predisposes them to a whole host of horrible chronic diseases. For these folks, changing their diets will be difficult but necessary in order to ensure long healthy lives. The easiest way to do this is slowly, one day at a time, rather than trying to do everything at once. For example, if you eat a lot of sugar, slowly cut down. Eat 1 dessert a day rather than 2. Add some extra veggies to your lunch and dinner. Changing your diet slowly will help you achieve your goal of eating the best diet possible.

Finally, we drink fresh water whenever possible. Filtered water helps reduce additional chemicals that may be found in the local water supply. Drinking large amounts of water to maintain hydration and encourage frequent eliminations (mainly via urination and secondarily bowel movements) helps remove toxins.

Chapter Lesson-You are what you eat. Your diet can keep you healthy or make you sick. It's often difficult for many people to make drastic, overnight changes to their diets. Therefore, make small changes over time and do what you can to eat fresh, preferably organic, foods whenever you can, minimizing processed foods that contain large amounts of sugar, high fructose corn syrup, chemical preservatives, and partially hydrogenated vegetable oils.

*Sandy's Thoughts: We are what we eat, and good diets as well as bad diets can regulate our genes and cause increased or decreased levels of inflammation in our bodies. Proper diet is the foundation of any treatment program regardless of whether you want to use natural therapies or conventional therapies. While I know that eating better can be challenging for many Americans, I encourage you to take little steps to improve your diet. Begin by eating a little less meat each day, then try to eat only 3-5 ounces of organic or natural meat no more than one meal per day. Try to eat more fresh cold water fish and fruits and vegetables. While I still enjoy the occasional dessert, and I was never a big sugar eater anyway, I have attempted to reduce my sugar intake as much as possible. Once again achieving the proper diet doesn't happen overnight and you shouldn't beat yourself up if it takes you a while to improve your diet or you occasionally indulge in a favorite food or meal. Do the best you can knowing that even a little progress can reduce your chances of your cancer returning.*

# Chapter 12

# *Understanding the Importance of Mind-Body Medicine*

*The power of prayer and other forms of mind-body medicine provide incredible healing, both physically and emotionally/spiritually, both for those with cancer and for those who offer support to cancer patients.*

*"Every woman who has breast cancer needs to look at the emotional conflict in her life."*

Stephen Sinatra, M.D., in *Knockout* by Suzanne Somers.

As there are many wonderful books that have been written exclusively on the topic of mind-body medicine, I will just keep my remarks in this chapter brief and to the point.

Mind-body medicine is an area of naturopathic medicine that recognizes the influence our minds and emotional states have on our bodies. We've all heard the term "psychosomatic" diseases. These are simply conditions where the body is negatively affected by adverse mental states. While the body is technically "ill" in people with psychosomatic disorders, the real problem is in the mind. Unless you treat the abnormal thought processes that are causing the body to react negatively, the body never will fully recover.

Note: Some doctors believe that their patients (particularly their female patients) are not suffering from true physical illnesses but rather simply believe that the illness is "all in their minds." These doctors unfortunately don't take the patient's complaints seriously, but they are not totally wrong. Diseases such as cancer can have a psychological or emotional component to them. By simply asking the patient "Tell me what's bothering you," doctors can uncover issues that may be the cause of the disease or at least contribute to a negative state of health that might impede true healing. True healing can only come about when the effects of the mind and emotions are recognized as contributing to the disease. This negative mental/emotional state must be treated in the same way that the physical disease is treated.

By recognizing the harmful influence negative emotions can have on our bodies, we can easily turn that thinking around and enjoy positive effects on our health if our minds and emotional states are functioning in a healthy manner.

Mind-body medicine makes use of techniques such as prayer, meditation, yoga, exercise, massage, rolfing, and music therapy. By using any or all of these techniques to reduce anxiety and unnecessary worry (all cancer patients, as well as their supportive family members, have anxieties and worries at various times in their diagnosis and treatment,) we can positively influence the health of the cancer patient. It's been well proven that a constant state of stress and anxiety and unnecessary worry create a whole host of problems in our bodies including a state of hypercortisolemia (too much cortisol is produced by the adrenal glands, which suppresses our immune systems,) excess epinephrine in our bloodstreams (which increases blood pressure and heart rate and decreases proper digestion and absorption of nutrients from the diet,) and insulin resistance (which predisposes people to obesity, type II diabetes, and cancer cell growth.)

Mind-body medicine techniques are designed to lower stress hormones in the patient's body and induce a sense of calmness. By returning to a calm physiological state our immune systems function better and cancer cells are less likely to grow and spread.

Additionally, studies have shown a positive benefit to women with Stage I, II, or III breast cancer who exercise, as physical activity after a breast cancer diagnosis may reduce the risk of death from this disease. The greatest benefit occurred in women who performed the equivalent of walking 3 to 5 hours per week at an average pace, with little evidence of a correlation between increased benefit and greater energy expenditure. Women with breast cancer (especially estrogen receptor positive cancers) who exercise may improve their survival.

Exercise may help the patient with cancer in several ways, including reducing breast density (in obese women,) improving physical and psychological health (improved quality of life with reduced stress,) and reducing chronic low-grade systemic inflammation (through the anti-inflammatory effects of exercise that are mediated by muscle-derived cytokines (myokines, specifically interleukin-6 which may reduce levels of tumor necrosis factor alpha.)

Finally, as a veterinarian, I obviously need to mention the positive benefits most people receive when sharing their lives with a special pet. Enjoying the companionship of a dog, cat, or really any pet can bring much joy to your life and lower your blood pressure and stress. If you have time to share your life with an animal, please do so as both you and your pet will receive numerous mind-body benefits.

It is the rare cancer doctor who discusses the positive and negative influences the mind and emotional states have on the cancer patient's body, yet it is important for you to find techniques that can help you deal with day-today stressors in order to maximize the benefits of whichever treatment you choose to fight your cancer. Working with a naturopathic doctor specializing in cancer can introduce you to the various mind-body techniques and allow you to determine which techniques are best suited to your desires.

Sandy has always exercised to stay healthy and keep her weight at an optimum weight. Since her cancer diagnosis she has added yoga and Pilates classes to her regimen. She continues to try to get a daily nap and goes for evening walks with me. By volunteering at our church she maintains a giving, selfless attitude and has positive interactions with other adults. Because Sandy believes several negative family events contributed to her diagnosis of breast cancer, the use of mind-body medicine is very important to her as she tries to live as stress-free a life as possible.

Chapter Lesson-By recognizing the negative influence bad emotional states can have on our bodies, we can easily turn that thinking around and enjoy positive effects on our health if our minds and emotional states are functioning in a healthy manner.

*Sandy's Thoughts: I believe stress is an overlooked but yet important cause of many diseases, including cancer. I believe my own cancer is a direct result of certain stressors in my life. Regular exercise, prayer, laughter, quality time spent with friends and family, and other mind-body medicine techniques are important to reduce your stress and allow you to take care of yourself. I also think it is important not to hold on to resentment or anger. It will manifest itself in muscle tension and soreness and cause inflammation, which if prolonged will lead to major health problems. It is so important to resolve any negative issues as soon as possible, especially while going through any treatments. Counseling is an effective tool to help with that.*

# Chapter 13

## *Using Supplements to Save Your Life*

*"As her husband, it's my role to be sure I always remember because I realize she will never forget."*

Anonymous

Unlike most other books on breast cancer, *Breast Choices for the Best Chances: Your Breasts, Your Life, and How You Can Win the Battle!* focuses on helping YOU make the best choice for YOU. A very important part of staying healthy and killing cancer involves the use of nutritional supplements. While there is a large volume of research showing the positive benefits of selected supplements in killing breast cancer cells, few conventional doctors have expertise in this area. Therefore, it is imperative that you work with a naturopathic doctor experienced in cancer.

IF you can't find a naturopathic doctor specializing in cancer therapy, I recommend the following resources:

*Life Extension Foundation* (www.lef.org)

This is an organization that is devoted to presenting scientifically valid information on the use of integrative medicine. The information is presented on its web site and monthly publication in language that is written for the (non-scientific) public, so it's very easy to understand. Members can purchase high quality supplements at very reasonable prices and also have access to lab tests at a reduced price, as well as being able to consult with naturopathic doctors. I highly recommend this organization.

*Cancer Treatment Centers of America*
(http://www.cancercenter.com/)

The Cancer Treatment Centers combine both conventional medical doctors and naturopathic doctors in the same facility, taking an integrative cancer treatment approach. In this manner, cancer patients can have all of their care under one roof. However, in Sandy's case, we knew we would get her conventional treatment done locally and instead spent a few days at our regional Cancer Treatment Center to gain a greater understanding of how to incorporate natural therapies into her treatment protocol.

*Oncology Association of Naturopathic Physicians*
(http://www.oncanp.org/)

This organization is composed of naturopathic doctors (and at least 1 naturopathic veterinarian-ME!) who have expressed interest in learning more about using natural therapies to treat people with cancer as the focus of their practices. I encourage you to consider one of their members to be your naturopathic doctor, as their members have expressed a special interest in the use of naturopathic therapies for the treatment of cancer.

The good news about using supplements to assist in the fight against cancer is that there are MANY supplements that can help you fight cancer, especially if you are a woman with early stage invasive breast cancer like Sandy and have decided not to use chemotherapy or tamoxifen. The bad news is that the use of supplements will result in an additional expense (our monthly supplement bill averaged $350 initially, but our maintenance supplement cost is about half of that) and insurance unfortunately will not reimburse you for the cost of the supplements. However, we feel the cost is minimal compared to the cost of traditional medical therapies, and fortunately we can afford the supplements so we don't have to place a cost on Sandy's life. We'll do as much as we can to keep her healthy and cancer-free. Another negative about the use of supplements is that the typical breast cancer patient will need to initially swallow about 50 capsules per day to get the maximum benefit from nutritional supplements.

Please don't be discouraged by the number of pills you need to take each day. Start slowly, with 1 or 2 supplements and do the best you can. Even just taking a few supplements each day will increase your chances of beating cancer and living a long healthy life.

*"No matter how much surgery you do to cut out cancer, or how much radiation you use to burn out cancer, or how much chemotherapy you use to poison cancer, if the patient's immune system is not functioning properly, that patient will die from cancer."*

That statement, made by world-famous cancer expert Dr. Russell Blaylock in my book, *The Natural Vet's Guide to Preventing and Treating Cancer in Dogs*, really says it all.

After surgery cuts out most of the cancer, and chemotherapy kills most of the cancer, and radiation burns most of the cancer, what's left to do destroy any remaining cancer cells, or to prevent another cancer from popping up in the future? Absolutely nothing! Unless the patient continues therapy, using a combination of proper diet, mind-body medicine, and nutritional supplements, any cancer cells that have survived conventional therapy will, at some point, continue to grow, spread, and ultimately kill the patient.

Unfortunately, unless you are familiar with naturopathic medicine or are lucky enough to work with a naturopathic doctor, your conventional doctors will not tell you any of this. Despite the fact that Sandy has visited several outstanding conventional doctors, not one of them, NOT ONE, has ever talked about the use of diet or supplements to kill cancer or boost her immune system to prevent a recurrence of her cancer.

The sad news is that so many cancer patients will ultimately die after surviving conventional therapies because nothing is done to prevent the recurrence of cancer. Ever since Sandy's diagnosis, it seems that not a day goes by that I don't discover that someone else I know has been diagnosed with cancer (usually breast cancer.) Often these cancers are caught at a stage where they are considered "curable." Yet not one of these patients is doing anything "natural" to support her immune system or continue the fight against cancer once conventional therapies are finished. How sad and tragic to know that many people will needlessly die out of ignorance once their cancer returns.

The most important reason I'm writing this book is to educate current and future cancer patients about all of their options. Just because your conventional doctors don't know about these options or don't agree with these options doesn't mean you shouldn't consider them.

Also keep in mind that the use of supplements is YOUR choice. Just because I believe in them and Sandy is using them to stay healthy and hopefully prevent future cancers doesn't mean that you will agree. This book is about choices, and while we both hope we can convince you of the need for lifelong immune support, the final choice about the use of nutritional supplements is still up to you.

To demonstrate just how strongly we feel about the use of natural therapies such as nutritional supplements, consider these questions: What are you doing now to make your conventional therapies more effective and reduce their side effects, and what will you do once you have finished your conventional cancer treatment to prevent your cancer from coming back?

Keep in mind that I am not suggesting that natural therapies are a cure-all. People are often diagnosed with cancer in very late stages, once it has spread throughout their bodies. For them, natural medicines can be an important part of managing their cancers even if a cure is not possible. For most people who are diagnosed with early stage cancer, however, integrating natural therapies with properly selected conventional therapies (or simply using natural therapies in place of conventional treatments) offers hope for a better outcome.

In this chapter, I will share with you the supplements that I have put together (with help from several naturopathic doctors) to help Sandy maximize the benefits from conventional therapies, reduce their side effects, and remain cancer-free the rest of her life. While there are no guarantees, we believe this is a better approach than simply doing nothing and waiting to see what happens (in most cases, depending upon the type of cancer and stage of cancer when it's first diagnosed, "what happens" is that the cancer returns and kills the patient.)

In my own veterinary practice, while I can never offer guarantees to my patients, I tell them that based upon my years of experience using natural therapies to help pets with cancer, I expect my patients to live one and a half to two times longer than their conventional doctors expect them to live IF they will use the natural therapies I have prescribed for them.

Please note that I am NOT saying that the supplements we have chosen for Sandy are appropriate for you if you have cancer. You MUST work with your naturopathic doctors to find the right treatments for you, similar to working with your conventional doctors to find the right conventional therapies for you.

It's never too early to start using doctor-supervised/prescribed nutritional supplements in your fight against cancer. While starting them at the time of diagnosis, prior to the use of any conventional therapies, is best, you can start them anytime, even if you've already completed surgery, chemotherapy, or radiation therapy, or if it has been many years since your initial diagnosis of cancer.

And since there are many out there who are skeptical about the effectiveness of natural supplements, I have included a description of why each supplement was chosen to help Sandy win the war against her cancer based upon volumes of research.

With rare exception, I have NOT listed the dosages of the supplements Sandy is taking. Supplements often function in a "drug-like" fashion, and the dosages vary based upon a variety of factors. Only your naturopathic doctor can determine which supplements and which dosages are most appropriate for you, and when possible (i.e., Vitamin D,) dosages should be based upon the results of your blood or urine testing.

Finally, keep in mind that nutritional supplements that are prescribed to help the woman with breast cancer function in the following ways: support/boost the immune system (by various mechanisms,) reduce inflammation (inflammation promotes cancer and many chronic diseases,) and modify estrogen (either by producing more of the "good" estrogen and less of the "bad" estrogen or by blocking estrogen's ability to stimulate cells to develop into cancer.)

Here then, is Sandy's supplement regimen (which changes depending upon her circumstances and as new research becomes available):

*Cimetidine*

Cimetidine is an antihistamine drug (H2 blocker) (rather than a true natural therapy) that is usually prescribed for its antacid function (blocking the production of stomach acid through inhibition of histamine's actions on the acid-secreting cells in the stomach.) However, it can be a safe drug when properly prescribed for short term use for cancer patients.

Taken at night before bed, it is very useful for cancer patients and works through several mechanisms of action: preventing suppression of the immune system caused by tumor secretion of histamine, halting cancer cell growth, preventing angiogenesis (new blood vessel formation that cancer cells need in order to grow and spread,) promoting cancer cell death (apoptosis,) and averting often fatal cancer metastasis (cimetidine inhibits cancer cell from sticking to each other, other tissues, and blood vessels by blocking the expression of an adhesive molecule called E-selectin on the surface of cells lining blood vessels. Cancer cells latch onto E-selectin in order to adhere to the lining of blood vessels; by preventing the expression of E-selectin, cimetidine significantly limits the ability of cancer cell adherence to the blood vessel walls.) Cimetidine also increases levels of important immune system cells called natural killer (NK) cells.

However, recent studies show that it may stimulate the hormone prolactin, which may stimulate the breast cells. In at least one study the administration of cimetidine to men decreased the 2-hydroxylation of estradiol (the less harmful form of estrogen) and resulted in an increase in the serum estradiol concentration. This mechanism may help to account for the signs and symptoms of estrogen excess reported with the long-term use of cimetidine. Because this could be harmful to women with estrogen receptor positive breast cancer, Sandy stopped taking cimetidine after several months of administration (she mainly took it around the time of her surgery when cancer cells are most likely to escape from the primary tumor due to handling of the tumor, and for 1 month following surgery.) Additionally, she is taking additional supplements which favor the formation of "good" estrogen (the 2-series) rather than "bad" estrogen (the 16 series) which are discussed in more detail in this chapter.

In at least one study, people taking cimetidine as part of their cancer treatment protocol tend to live longer than patients who do not take cimetidine (improved 10 year survival rate.)

*NSAIDS*

NSAIDs, specifically aspirin, may lower serum estradiol levels and inhibit NF kappa B. Aspirin seems to be helpful in women with either ER-positive or ER-negative tumors.

Aspirin use could possibly increase survival among women with breast cancer as it inhibits production of prostaglandins and cyclooxygenase via inhibition of COX-1 and COX-2 enzymes. Studies have shown that breast cancers produce prostaglandins in greater amounts than normal breast cells and that aspirin can inhibit the growth and decrease the invasiveness of breast cancer cells. It can also reduce cytokines that are involved in the spread of cancer cells to bones and also stimulate immune response. Finally, aspirin may help reduce the spread of cancer by preventing the dilation of lymphatic vessels. A major study reported a survival advantage among women with breast cancer who take aspirin: there was a decreased risk of distant recurrence, breast cancer death, and death from any cause. The current recommendation is to take low doses of aspirin (1 baby aspirin, enteric- coated if possible to reduce GI irritation) 5 days per week to achieve maximum effects.

*Melatonin*

While well-known as a sleep aid, high dose melatonin is prescribed for patients with cancer due to its effect as an anti-oxidant (particularly in neutralizing the hydroxyl radical.) It is also effective in reducing adverse effects of as well as enhancing the cancer killing ability of various chemotherapy drugs. For breast cancer patients, administering melatonin with tamoxifen may increase the effectiveness of and reduce side effects of tamoxifen. Melatonin may also directly modulate estrogen receptor expression to inhibit breast cancer cell growth (especially valuable in the most common form of breast cancer: ER-positive tumors) and also boosts the production of immune components that kill metastasized cancer cells. Sandy used this for a few months following her diagnosis and surgery, then stopped it since her cancer was "cured" and she had decided not to take tamoxifen.

*Detoxification*

Sandy has used 2 methods of detoxification as part of her treatment protocol.

She started with a mild homeopathic detoxification using the Detox Kit from Heel. These remedies are designed to gently cleanse the body, and are helpful at the time of cancer diagnosis and for support during conventional therapies. She also took their homeopathic mistletoe medication (*Viscum album*) for the first month following her diagnosis as it is recommended as a therapy for people with cancer.

The second method involves the daily administration of the herb milk thistle. Milk thistle, occasionally called Holy Thistle or St. Mary's Thistle, contains silymarin, which contains three major flavolignans: silibinin (silybin,) silidyanin, and silychristin, as well as other compounds such as apigenin, histamine, oleic acid, stearic acid, palmitic acid, and myristic acid.

Silymarin has been shown to protect the liver from damage by various chemicals and functions as a liver-protective supplement by altering the outer liver cell membrane so that toxins cannot enter the cell. Silymarin inhibits the growth of certain human cancer lines in vitro and inhibits the 5-LOX pathway, reducing inflammation in the body. Silymarin also functions as an antioxidant.

Silymarin also fights cancer by inhibiting intestinal beta-glucoronidase, modulating carcinogen metabolizing enzymes, and inhibiting epidermal growth factor receptor and kinases.

*Green Tea*

Green tea is a very popular supplement used to assist in the treatment of cancer. Epigallocatechin gallate (EGCG) is the most powerful of the catechins contained in green and black tea and functions as an antioxidant that is about 25-100 times more potent than vitamins C and E.

EGCG has a number of benefits to help the patient with cancer, including: suppresses angiogenesis (new blood vessel growth that tumors use to grow and spread;) helps prevent metastasis in a number of ways, including inhibiting the secretion of collagenases by tumor cells, thus arresting their ability to invade normal tissue; enhancing glucuronization of estrogens in the liver, a process through which estrogens are rendered inactive by being conjugated with glucuronic acid, into a form in which they are excreted from the body (very important in preventing and treating breast cancer;) protects against radiation-induced DNA damage (possibly by scavenging the dangerous hydroxyl radical that is formed by radiation damage to the cell;) inhibits the activation of protein kinase C, and interferes with the binding of growth factors to their receptors (in the case of breast cancer, catechins interfere with the binding of estrogen to estrogen receptors;) inhibits the release of tumor necrosis factor alpha (TNF-alpha), a highly inflammatory cytokine, and of nitric oxide synthase, an enzyme necessary for the production of nitric oxide (nitric oxide plays an important role in inflammation and carcinogenesis;) inhibits telomerase (the enzyme that keeps cancer cells alive by maintaining the end portions of the tumor cell chromosomes.)

In the presence of EGCG, cancer cells (but not normal cells) exhibited telomere shortening and death. EGCG interferes with the enzyme NOX (NOX, an enzyme is required for growth by both normal and malignant cells. While normal cells express NOX only when dividing, tumor cells express it all the time. The tumor form of the enzyme is called t-NOX, or tumor-associated NOX. Drugs that inhibit t-NOX also inhibit tumor growth. EGCG inhibits t-NOX while sparing the NOX of healthy cells;) lowers serum glucose and insulin (elevated insulin is a potent growth factor for many kinds of tumors, and also is a pro-inflammatory and immunosuppressive hormone, the lowering of insulin in itself should help prevent cancer or, in cases of existing cancer, slow down its growth;) and protects the liver against damage during tamoxifen administration.

EGCG arrests tumor cell growth in a different cell-cycle stage than curcumin; EGCG in green tea arrests cancer cell growth at the G1 phase. When the two compounds are combined, growth inhibition was enhanced, suggesting a synergistic effect.

*Curcumin (Turmeric)*

Curcumin, the active ingredient in the spice turmeric, significantly lowers the expression of the MDR1 gene. This gene controls a cellular "pump" which is responsible for removing toxins, including chemotherapy drugs, from cells. When curcumin lowers the expression of the MDR1 gene, the P-glycoprotein pump of cancer cells is inhibited, which can increase the effectiveness of chemotherapy as the cancer cells can't easily "pump" the drugs out of the cells before the cells die.

Curcumin is also a potent antioxidant that is best known for its use during radiation therapy where it increases the effectiveness of radiation as well as reduces side effects of radiation therapy. Curcumin (like the drug tamoxifen) also blocks access of estrogen to cells and protects against chemicals that mimic estrogen (like estrogen, manmade estrogen-mimicking chemicals called xenoestrogens that are plentiful in our environment promote the growth of breast cancer.) In a study on human breast cancer cells, curcumin reversed growth caused by 17b-estradiol by 98%. The toxic chemical DDT's growth-enhancing effects on breast cancer were blocked about 75% by curcumin.

Curcumin also inhibits multiple kinase enzymes that are necessary for cancer cell growth and spread. Curcumin, known for its anti-inflammatory action, inhibits cyclooxygenase (COX) and lipoxygenase (LOX), two enzymes that promote inflammation. Inflammation plays significant and diverse roles in the initiation and promotion of cancer.

Curcumin arrests the growth of cancer cells in the G2 stage and induces apoptosis (death) of cancer cells. Combining EGCG (which arrests cancer cell growth at the G1 phase) with curcumin increases the odds of killing more cells.

Curcumin blocks AP-1, thereby decreasing angiogenesis (new blood vessel growth is needed for tumors to grow and spread.)

Curcumin's effects are a dose dependent response, and a standardized product is essential.

Sandy is taking a specialized type of curcumin called Super BioCurcumin by Life Extension. This product allows a lower dose to be taken (fewer capsules per day) yet achieves the same bioavailability as "regular" curcumin.

*Quercetin*

Quercetin, another powerful antioxidant, suppresses cell proliferation, promotes programmed cell death (apoptosis,) and protects DNA.

Quercetin, **especially when combined with curcumin** (another antioxidant with anti-inflammatory and tumor-blocking potential,) minimizes damage in tissues exposed to radiation (mammography) while increasing the cancer killing ability of radiation (such as radiation received with breast cancer radiation treatment.)

*Resveratrol*

Resveratrol exhibits many anti-cancer properties, including suppression of tumor growth by increasing or decreasing the production of various enzymes and molecules that regulate cellular reproduction and blood supply to the tumor. Through these mechanisms, resveratrol may enhance the anti-cancer effects of chemotherapeutic drugs and radiation. With its potent antioxidant capabilities, resveratrol may even protect healthy tissues from damage induced by chemotherapy.

*Astaxanthin*

Astaxanthin, the pigment that is the most commonly occurring red carotenoid in marine and aquatic animals, is a potent antioxidant and anti-inflammatory supplement. Astaxanthin is produced by the microalgae *Haematoccous pluvialis.* There are two main sources of astaxanthin: the microalgae that produce it and the animals that eat the algae (salmon, shellfish, and krill).

Astaxanthin is now thought to be the most powerful antioxidant found in nature, even more powerful that other well-known antioxidants such as beta-carotene, alpha-tocopherol, lycopene, and lutein. While many naturopaths recommend astaxanthin, there are no studies on its use in treating breast cancer per se (although it has been shown to inhibit cancer cell growth of various cancers in the lab.) Astaxanthin also regulates genes involved in cancer cell growth and communication and stimulates production of interleukin-1 and tumor necrosis factor to help kill cancer cells. It is used due to its anti-inflammatory and antioxidant activity but more studies are needed in breast cancer patients to determine the "best dose" to use.

*Flax/Lignans*

Flaxseed is the richest source of lignans (providing up to 800 times more than any other plant) and alpha linolenic acid (ALA.) Lignans are both antioxidants (compounds that protect cells from oxidative damage) and phytoestrogens (weak plant estrogens that inhibit the body's own harmful estrogen and protect breast cells from developing cancer.) Lignans have been shown to inhibit the growth and spread of breast cancer cells, possibly due to down-regulation of insulin-like growth factor I and epidermal growth factor receptor expression. In one study of 1122 post-menopausal women with breast cancer, higher intake of lignans significantly reduced breast cancer mortality. Although the dietary intake of lignans did not have any effect on breast cancer survival in premenopausal women, postmenopausal women with a high intake of plant lignans were approximately 70% less likely to die from their breast cancer. While Sandy is premenopausal, she has decided to take flax anyway since it can't hurt, it certainly has health benefits, she will be menopausal within a few years, and possibly it will reduce the chances of new tumors developing while she is still premenopausal.

Ground flax seed (but not flax oil) provides a healthy dose of lignans. The most efficient way of consuming fresh flax seed with other cancer-fighting phytochemicals is to consume 2-5 tablespoons a day of freshly ground brown (or golden) flax seeds (grind the seeds every few days and keep them refrigerated to prevent oxidation of the flax oil in the seeds that can occur with "aging" ground flax seed.)

Research indicates that higher blood levels of enterolactone, the primary lignan made by the body from flaxseed, are associated with a lower risk of breast cancer. Conversely, values of serum enterolactone were significantly lower in women who subsequently developed breast cancer, leading researchers to conclude that the phytoestrogen enterolactone had a strong protective effect on breast cancer risk.

Lignans also have non-hormonal actions including antioxidant and antiangiogenic effects. Studies have shown significant reductions in breast cancer risk in women with the highest versus the lowest quartile of urinary enterolactone excretion, serum enterolactone levels, or lignan intake. Flaxseed also has a high concentration of α-linolenic acid which has been shown in animal and human studies to be protective against breast cancer.

It has been suggested that the lignans act as anti-estrogens by competing with estradiol for binding to the estrogen receptor. Enterolactone has also been shown to inhibit the activity of aromatase, leading to a reduction of endogenous estrogen synthesis (the aromatase enzyme is responsible for synthesizing estrogen, and many women with breast cancer are prescribed aromatase-enzyme inhibiting drugs.)

For women with ER-positive breast cancer who choose to take tamoxifen, studies have shown that, at least in the short-term, flaxseed enhances the effectiveness of tamoxifen in reducing tumor growth, both in the presence of high and low levels of estrogen; studies have also shown that invasiveness and adhesiveness of human tumor cells are reduced to a greater extent by the lignans in combination with tamoxifen than by either one alone.

Lignans may also protect against endometrial cancer, a condition associated with prolonged exposure to unopposed estrogens. Flax lignans may offer protection through an anti-estrogenic effect in the body. Researchers in California assessed lignan intake and cancer status among nearly 1,000 women in the San Francisco area and determined that women with the highest dietary lignan intake experienced the lowest risk of developing this carcinoma of the uterine lining (note that endometrial cancer is a well-known but rare side effect of tamoxifen therapy; women taking tamoxifen should also consider taking flax seeds.)

It is suggested that there are several ways that lignans may reduce breast cancer: decreased estrogen production (by blocking the aromatase enzyme;) by blocking the estrogen receptors in the breast from stronger cancer-stimulating estrogens in a similar way tamoxifen works; by preferentially creating more "good" estrogen (increasing levels of 2-hydroxyestrone rather than the more harmful 16-hydroxyestrone;) by making breast tissue more resistant to the damaging effects of environmental toxins; by increasing well-differentiated breast tissue which is more resistant to damage; by inhibiting the growth of breast cancer cells; by decreasing the incidence of metastasis; by decreasing levels of VEGF (which reduces blood vessel growth to the cancer cells;) and by lengthening the menstrual cycle (the more menstrual cycles a woman has the greater the risk of breast cancer due to increased estrogen exposure.)

Flaxseeds contain over 300,000 mcg lignans/100 grams. In one study, the lowest risk of dying was seen in women consuming >318 mcg per day; in another study, those women in the highest quartile of total lignan intake (>1395 µg/day) had a reduced risk of breast cancer. High dietary intakes of plant lignans and high exposure to enterolignans were associated with reduced risks of ER positive and PR positive postmenopausal breast cancer in a Western population that did not consume a diet rich in soy. In addition to flax seed, lignans can be consumed in other food products including: curly kale (2321 mcg/100 grams,) broccoli (1325 mcg,) white cabbage (787 mcg,) brussel sprouts (747 mcg,) sauerkraut (316 mcg,) red cabbage (276 mcg,) cauliflower (185 mcg,) garlic (536 mcg,) apricots (450 mcg,) strawberries (334 mcg,) peaches (293 mcg,) pears (193 mcg,) nectarines (190 mcg,) raisins, white (181 mcg,) raisins, blue (144 mcg,) grapefruit, pink (152 mcg,) cherries (147 mcg,) kiwi (129 mcg.)

*Fish Oil*

Omega-3 fatty acids, most commonly found in high amounts in cold water fish such as salmon and tuna (and some nuts such as walnuts and flax,) reduce inflammation in the body and help breast cancer patients in a number of ways.

One study examining levels of fatty acids in breast adipose tissue of breast cancer patients has shown that pro-inflammatory omega-6 fatty acids may be contributing to the high risk of breast cancer in the United States and that omega-3 fatty acids, derived from fish oil, may have a protective effect.

A higher omega-3:omega-6 ratio may reduce the risk of breast cancer, especially in premenopausal women.

Omega-3 fatty acids (primarily eicosapentanoic acid (EPA) and docosahexaneoic acid (DHA)) have been shown to retard the growth of breast cancer in the lab and in animal experiments, and inhibit tumor development and metastasis (spread.)

Fish oils have anti-proliferative effects at high doses, reducing the growth of cancer cells.

When breast cancer cells are exposed to the omega-3 fatty acids EPA and DHA, cancer cell apoptosis (self-destruction/death) increases. EPA and DHA inhibit the pro-inflammatory enzyme cyclooxygenase 2 (COX 2,) an enzyme that leads to inflammation and therefore promotes breast cancer. Omega-3's activate a cell membrane receptor called peroxisome proliferator-activated receptor (PPAR,), which is a key regulator of lipid (fat) metabolism but is also capable of shutting down proliferative/growth activity in many of cells including breast cells. Omega-3's increase the expression of two tumor suppressor genes, BRCA1 and BRCA2. When functioning normally, these genes help repair damage to DNA, thus helping to prevent cancer development.

When researchers examined the expression of BRCA1 and BRCA2 in breast cell lines after treatment with both omega-6 and omega-3 fats, they found that EPA and DHA induced increases in BRCA1 and BRCA2, but omega-6 fats, found in meat and dairy products and oils such as corn and safflower oil, did not.

While some cases of breast cancer arise from genetic factors (about 5% of cases are due to mutations in BRCA 1 and 2,) most are linked to diet, lifestyle, and exposure to environmental triggers. Studies suggest that chronic activation of a pro-inflammatory gene switch (transcription factor) called Nf-KappaB is important to cancer cell survival. NFKB has also been found to play important roles in all stages of breast cancer development. A study using female breast cells shows that omega-3 fatty acids from fish oil suppress activation of NFKB.

Fish oil in the diet was also found to significantly increase the level of PTEN protein in the breast tumors (PTEN is a tumor suppressor gene which has been shown to be important in the inhibition of the development of cancer.)

Additionally fish oil reduces PI 3 kinase and Akt kinase activity in breast tumors (leading to significant inhibition of NFκB activation) and prevents the expression of the anti-apoptotic proteins Bcl-2 and Bcl-XL in the breast tumors.

## Tips for increasing Omega-3 and decreasing Omega-6 fats in your diet:

Add walnuts to salads, muffins and cereal, and snack on nuts and dried fruit instead of crackers or processed foods.

Add 2-4 tablespoons of ground flaxseed to your food (cereal, oatmeal, yogurt, etc.) daily.

Cook with canola, olive, peanut or walnut oil instead of vegetable, corn or soybean oil (note:canola oil, and other oils, may be prepared from genetically modified seeds which have been noted by some naturopaths as possibly contributing to health problems, including cancer. Olive oil would be a better choice than canola oil.)

Replace store-bought salad dressings (often made with soybean or other "inflammatory" oils) with homemade dressings made with olive oil and flavored (balsamic, etc.) vinegar.

Eat FRESH (not farmed) cold water fish at least 1-2 times weekly, with an emphasis on wild salmon.

Choose natural or organic eggs that say "high in omega-3" which come from chickens that eat flaxseed. More omega-3 is deposited in the egg yolk, making them a rich source of this beneficial fat.

Avoid foods with hydrogenated or partially hydrogenated oils as these are pro-inflammatory.

## Krill Oil

Recently many naturopathic doctors have been recommending krill oil, given with or sometimes in place of fish oil.

Krill oil is made from krill, small, shrimp-like crustaceans, and like fish oil, contains the omega-3 fatty acids EPA and DHA. However, in fish oil, these omega-3 fats are found in the triglyceride form. In krill oil, they are found in a double chain phospholipid structure. The fats in human cell membranes are in the phospholipid form. The phospholipid structure of the EPA and DHA in krill oil is reported to make them much more absorbable. Krill oil also contains vitamin E, vitamin A, vitamin D and astaxanthin, which is a potent anti-oxidant.

While there is much less research on the use of krill oil in treating breast cancer, it is worth discussing this topic with your naturopathic doctor.

## Olive Oil

Oleuropein from olive fruit has additional biological properties including enhancement of antioxidant mechanisms. Diets high in monosaturated oils such as olive oil are also less inflammatory as these diets contain less pro-inflammatory fats (omega 6 fatty acids, partially hydrogenated oils, etc.)

Those afflicted with certain inherited genetic mutations are predisposed to contracting disorders related to defects in cell reproduction. A gene of particular concern to some women is HER2, and in studies oleuropein effectively down-regulated HER2 expression. It is theorized that this may be one reason why those who eat a Mediterranean diet high in olive oil have such marked reductions in disorders like breast cancer that can be related to excess expression of the HER2 gene.

Sandy and I routinely use olive oil throughout the day, for cooking (such as our organic brown eggs for breakfast,) as part of our homemade salad dressing, and with aged balsamic vinegar/freshly ground black pepper (which has its own health benefits including antioxidant/antibacterial/gastrointestinal supporting activities) and freshly grown herbs for making bruschetta or simply as a dipping sauce for freshly made bread.

*CLA (Conjugated Linoleic Acid)*

CLA has direct breast cancer cell inhibitory effects. CLA has been shown both in the lab and in animal models to have strong anti-tumor activity. One study which examined the effect of dietary CLA on the growth of human breast adenocarcinoma cells in mice showed that dietary CLA inhibited local tumor growth by 73% and 30% at nine and 14 weeks post-inoculation, respectively. Moreover, CLA completely stopped the spread of breast cancer cells to the lungs, bloodstream, and bone marrow.

*Coenzyme Q-10*

Blood levels of coenzyme Q10 are frequently reduced in cancer patients. In several small studies, positive results were seen in patients taking anywhere from 90 mg per day up to 300-400 mg per day. In some of the patients, complete regression of their residual breast tumors occurred. All breast cancer patients who supplemented with CoQ10 experienced decreased use of painkillers, improved quality of life, and an absence of weight loss.

Coenzyme Q10 may be useful in treating cancer because it boosts the immune system. Also, studies suggest that CoQ10 may prevent the growth of cancer cells directly. As an antioxidant, coenzyme Q10 may help prevent cancer from developing.

Data suggests that CoQ10 may also help fight cancer by significantly reducing expression of the bcl-2 gene family, which is responsible for conferring resistance to cell death. CoQ10 modulates bcl-2 in a manner that allows the cancer cells to kill themselves without harming normal cells.

*Vitamin D3*

*"75% of breast cancer could be prevented with higher vitamin D serum levels."*

Dr. Cedric F. Garland of the Moores Cancer Center and UCSD School of Medicine.

Research shows that most people are severely deficient in Vitamin D, even those who receive sunlight exposure. It is recommended that vitamin D3 (not vitamin D2, the form often prescribed by doctors) should be a supplement most people take for its numerous health benefits, including cancer prevention.

Optimizing vitamin D levels may be one of the most important steps you can take to stay healthy; in fact, vitamin D is not simply a vitamin but also a neuroregulatory hormone that influences nearly 3,000 different genes in your body.

Vitamin D kills cancer by promoting cell differentiation and supporting apoptosis (normal programmed cell death), as well as helping to prevent metastases and angiogenesis (new blood vessel formation needed for cancer to grow and spread.)

Increased mammographic density is considered a strong risk factor for breast cancer. Women who had a combined daily intake of 100 IU or more of Vitamin D combined with 750 mg or more of calcium demonstrated decreased breast density compared to women with lower intakes of the two nutrients, suggesting that adequate consumption of Vitamin D and calcium may reduce breast cancer risk.

Vitamin D3 works synergistically with tamoxifen to inhibit breast cancer cell proliferation.

Compared with sun-deprived women, women from lower, sunnier latitudes typically have lower rates of breast cancer. Additionally, the women from sunny places who consumed the most dietary vitamin D (from foods and supplements) enjoyed a greater breast-risk reduction than the women who consumed less dietary vitamin D (a combination of ample sun exposure and ample vitamin D intake was associated with the greatest risk reduction, compared with getting vitamin D from either sunlight or diet alone.) In general, 30 minutes of daily sun exposure creates 10,000 IU of Vitamin D3 in your body.

The Food & Nutrition Board of the U.S. Institute of Medicine just tripled the recommended daily allowances for vitamin D3 from 200 IU for adults to 600 IU. However, most naturopathic physicians recommend a minimum of 1000 IU per day and many are now recommending at least 8000 IU per day in order to raise blood levels to at least 50-70 ng/ml, considered an optimal or normal level for healthy people (Sandy is taking 17,000 IU per day;

the ideal amount should be based upon blood testing for vitamin D levels.) For cancer patients, a target goal for Vitamin D3 blood levels should be at least 60-80 ng/ml and maybe even closer to 80-100 ng/ml (most people have levels less than 35, with 35 being a minimum level for health.) New research shows that even higher daily doses of oral vitamin D3 (10,000-50,000 IU/day) are unlikely to be associated with toxicity (defined as blood levels above 200 ng/ml.) However, the best dose for each person to reach a target range of at least 60-80 ng/ml (and a range of 80-100 ng/ml for cancer patients) is best determined by blood testing due to individual response to supplemental vitamin D3.

Because vitamin K and iodine are also important for breast cancer patients (iodine deficiency has been linked to increased risks of breast cancer, and iodine supplementation provides additional iodine that can decrease the ability of estrogen to bind to estrogen receptors on the breast cells,) the vitamin D3 supplement Sandy takes from Life Extension also contains iodine and vitamin K. If you suffer from thyroid problems or take thyroid hormone, check with your doctor before supplementing with iodine to make sure it's safe to do so.

Finally, keep in mind that vitamin D is a fat soluble vitamin. This means that it is not only stored in your body but that its absorption in the intestinal tract is increased if taken with a fatty (rather than a high fiber) meal or with 1 to 2 teaspoons of a healthy fats such as olive oil.

*Modified Citrus Pectin (MCP)*

As discussed in the chapter on surgery, research indicates that MCP significantly increases the urinary excretion of toxic heavy metals like aluminum and mercury and inhibits tumor growth and metastasis.

MCP works by interacting with specialized proteins called galectins. MCP may help fight certain cancers by binding with galectin-3 to help decrease cancer cell aggregation, adhesion, and metastasis.

Galactose-binding lectins (galectins) are carbohydrate-binding proteins detected within some cancer cells (especially breast and colon cancer cells, and melanoma and prostate cancer cells) that help the cells clump together more easily and then attach to the inner linings of blood vessels. The adherence of these circulating tumor cells to the blood vessel walls is an essential step for the process of metastasis. This may facilitate the growth and spread of certain types of cancer. Galectin-3 may be particularly important in numerous processes involved in cancer, such as cancer adhesion, migration, progression, and metastasis. MCP may also increase apoptotic responses of tumor cells to chemotherapy (increasing tumor cell death when exposed to chemotherapy) by inhibiting galectin-3 anti-apoptotic function (tumor cells use various substances to resist chemotherapy, including galactin-3; by inhibiting galactin-3, MCP increases the effectiveness of chemotherapy.) Finally, MCP can inhibit angiogenesis (new blood vessel growth) which is critical for tumor growth and spread. Due to its anti-adhesive, apoptosis-promoting, and apoptosis-inducing properties, MCP can target multiple critical steps involved in cancer metastasis and may dramatically increase the effectiveness conventional chemotherapy.

Increased levels of galectin-3 in the blood or tissue are associated with more frequent cancer metastasis or an increased stage of tumor progression. Other findings suggest that intracellular galectin-3 exerts an anti-apoptotic effect, protecting cancer cells against programmed cell death by affecting mitochondrial function.

Taking MCP prior to, at the time of, and immediately following surgery can help reduce the spread of cancer cells that consistently occurs when tumors are manipulated. Sandy took MCP prior to her surgery and for about 3 months following the surgery.

*Mushroom Extracts (Beta Glucans/PSK)*

Medicinal mushrooms contain a number of active ingredients including polysaccharides and protein complexes including beta glucans. These ingredients may help the breast cancer patient by inhibiting NF-κB activity (NF-κB is involved in inflammation, cell survival, and transformation of normal cells into cancer cells.) A number of mushrooms have shown positive effects in treating patients with cancer including *Ganoderma lucidum, Agaricus bisporus, Agaricus blazei , A. brasiliensis, Trametes versicolor, Grifola frondosa, Inonotus obliquus, Lentinus edodes, Leucoagaricus americanus, Pleurotus ostreatus, Sparassis crispa, Cordyceps sinensis*, and *Coriolus versicolor.*

Mushrooms inhibit cell proliferation and cell cycle arrest at the G2/M phase of highly invasive human breast cancer cells and inhibit the expression of cell cycle regulatory genes (ANAPC2, ANAPC2, BIRC5, Cyclin B1, Cyclin H, CDC20, CDK2, CKS1B, Cullin 1, E2F1, KPNA2, PKMYT1 and TFDP1.) Mushrooms also suppress metastasis inhibiting cell adhesion, cell migration, and cell invasion.

PSK (protein-bound polysaccharide K) is a specially prepared extract from *Coriolus versicolor* that can increase natural killer cell (NK cell) and interleukin-1 and 2 activity and suppresses tumor cell invasiveness by down-regulating several invasion-related factors. Additional studies have shown that PSK inhibits the ability of cancer cells to form new blood vessels (angiogenesis) in mice. Cancer patients (various cancer types) taking PSK supplements had clinically significantly greater 5 year survival than those patients not taking this supplement.

Sandy was taking a *Maitake* mushroom supplement at the start of her cancer treatment. However, her naturopathic doctor switched her to a *Coriolus* mushroom supplement as it was felt that there was greater clinical data supporting the advantages of this particular mushroom supplement.

*Indole-3-Carbinol (I3C, Cruciferous Vegetables)/ Green Food Extract-Cruciferous Vegetables*

Indole-3-carbinol (I3C,) a product of glucosinolates present in cruciferous vegetables, is a potent inducer of liver cytochrome P450 enzymes. A protective effect may occur due to increased 2-hydroxylation and consequent inactivation of endogenous estrogens. I3C appears to be effective in shifting the metabolism of estradiol from the dangerous 16-alpha-hydroxylase pathway to the 2-hydroxylase pathway. As a result, consumption of I3C boosts the ratio of 2-OHE1:16a-OHE1, which correlates with reduced risk of breast and other cancers, including cervical, prostate, and even head and neck cancers. Cruciferous vegetable compounds (such as I3C) are effective in shifting estrogen metabolism to the more beneficial pathway, thus reducing levels of toxic 16-alpha-hydroxyestrone and increasing levels of protective 2-hydroxyestrone.

I3C also lowers the expression of metalloproteinase-9, an enzyme associated with breast cancer's invasiveness, and I3C lowers production of pro-inflammatory chemicals such as nitric oxide (NO) and prostaglandins (PGE.)

I3C induces degradation of Cdc25A, arrest of the $G_1$ phase of the cancer cell cycle, and inhibition of the growth of breast cancer cells.

Dietary intake of I3C reduces the development of estrogen-enhanced cancers, including breast, endometrial, and cervical cancers. While estrogen increases the growth and survival of tumors, I3C has been found to cause decreased growth and increased apoptosis (programmed cell death).

I3C also: increases the conversion of estradiol to the safer estriol; inhibits the growth of estrogen-receptor-positive breast cancer cells by 90% (compared to tamoxifen's 60%) by stopping the cell cycle; prevents chemically-induced breast cancer in rodents by 70-96%; acts as an antoixidant to inhibit free radicals (particularly those that cause the oxidation of fat;) stops the synthesis of DNA by about 50% in estrogen-receptor-negative cells, whereas tamoxifen had no significant effect; restores p21 and other proteins that act as checkpoints during the synthesis of a new cancer cell (tamoxifen has no effect on p21;) and reduces DNA damage in breast cells by 91%.

According to information from Life Extension Foundation, I3C controls estrogen metabolism through the same receptor that allows dioxin into the cell (the "Ah" receptor (aryl hydrocarbon)). Ah is similar to the estrogen receptor in that it can induce cellular growth. Unlike the estrogen receptor, however, scientists haven't found the body's natural "Ah" that fits into the Ah receptor. The only substances known to activate Ah are certain phytochemicals, including I3C-and the proven cancer promoter, dioxin (a very toxic chemical made from chlorine that is used in many things such as plastic food wrap/pesticides/wood preservatives, and concentrated in foods such as meat/dairy products/fish. Because it resides in fat, it's almost impossible to remove from the human body.)

The toxic chemical dioxin, like I3C, affects estrogen metabolism. For this reason, it has been called an estrogen blocker (like tamoxifen). Dioxin and I3C both affect estrogen metabolism through the Ah receptor. In addition to changing the metabolism of estrogen, dioxin also disrupts other important growth regulatory factors.

Among those factors are insulin, IGF-1 (insulin-like growth factor), and tumor necrosis factor (TNF). It also activates cancer genes and suppresses tumor suppressor genes.

I3C, on the other hand, fits into the Ah receptor, but instead of sending signals that help cancer grow, it sends signals that stop cancer growth. I3C uses the Ah receptor to indirectly affect estrogen metabolism also, but in a beneficial way and also it can also keep dioxin out of cells. When researchers at Texas A & M University treated breast cancer cells with I3C and dioxin at the same time, dioxin's adverse effects were reduced 90% by I3C.

In estrogen receptor-negative cells I3C stopped the synthesis of DNA for new cells by about 50% whereas tamoxifen had no significant effect. A study on rodents shows that damaged DNA in breast cells is reduced 91% by I3C.

While there is no proven breast cancer preventive, the most comprehensive scientific evidence so far stands behind phytochemicals such as I3C, which beat out more than 80 other substances, **including tamoxifen**, for anti-cancer potential in an assay done at the National Cancer Institute.

Caution: Pregnant women should not take I3C because of its modulation of estrogen. I3C appears to act both at the ovarian and hypothalamic levels, whereas tamoxifen appears to act only on the hypothalamic-pituitary axis as an anti-estrogen. Both I3C and tamoxifen block ovulation by altering preovulatory concentrations of luteinizing hormone (LH) and follicle stimulating hormone (FSH.) The reported aversion to cruciferous vegetables by pregnant women may be associated with their ability to change estrogen metabolism. Estrogen is a necessary growth factor for the fetus.

Other compounds in cruciferous vegetables which have shown cancer fighting ability (and which are often included in cruciferous vegetable supplements) include apigenin, benzyl isothiocyanate (BITC,) sulforaphane, and diindolylmethane (DIM.) A combination of these compounds offers the greatest promise for the prevention and many cancers as they act at multiple stages in the formation of cancer.

*Whey Protein* (Ideally Organic Whey Protein, which is obtained from dairy cows that have not been treated with growth hormones and antibiotics)

Whey appears to inhibit the growth of breast cancer cells when taken even at low concentrations (30 grams per day.) Whey protein concentrate selectively depletes cancer cells of their glutathione, thus making them more susceptible to cancer treatments such as radiation and chemotherapy. The concentration of glutathione in tumor cells is higher than that of the normal cells that surround them, and this difference in glutathione concentration may be an important factor in cancer cells' resistance to chemotherapy (an increase in glutathione concentration in cancer cells appears to be at least one of the mechanisms of acquired drug resistance to chemotherapy.)

Depletion of cancer cell glutathione decreases the rate of cellular proliferation and inhibits cancer growth. It's difficult to reduce glutathione sufficiently in tumor cells without placing healthy tissue at risk and putting the cancer patient in a worse condition. Whey protein can selectively deplete the cancer cells of their glutathione while increasing, or at least maintaining, the levels of glutathione in healthy cells.

In research it has been found that cancer cells exposed to whey proteins were depleted of their glutathione and their growth was inhibited, while normal cells had an increase in glutathione and increased cellular growth.

Sandy enjoys using organic whey protein in her daily shakes, both as part of her cancer therapy and as a nutritious "meal" following her work-outs in the morning.

*What About Soy?*

You'll notice that soy is missing from the list of Sandy's supplements. That's because the research on the benefits of soy in women with breast cancer is conflicting. While some studies have shown decreased growth of breast cancer cells exposed to soy extracts, other studies have shown enhanced growth of breast cancer cells exposed to soy extracts (and in some studies there was a negation of the positive effects of tamoxifen in blocking estrogen receptors on ER + cells, enhancing their growth.)

Another side effect of large amounts of soy includes increased levels of glutamate, a nervous system toxin.

Additionally, many people take proteolytic pancreatic enzymes, the main anti-cancer element of a cancer program developed by well-known cancer doctor Nick Gonzalez. Soy is well known for its ability to neutralize these proteolytic pancreatic enzymes, rendering them ineffective in the treatment of cancer.

Finally, in a study comparing the effects of flaxseed, soy, and placebo on the formation of the safer 2-hydroxyestrone estrogen metabolite (versus 16-hydroxyestrone,) it was shown that dietary supplementation with 25 grams of flaxseed significantly altered estrogen metabolism to a greater extent than that seen with the same amount of soy in postmenopausal women, and that this may have antiestrogenic effect by increasing the proportion of less biologically active estrogen, 2-hydroxyestrone relative to the estrogenic 16-hydroxyestrone, due to the higher lignan content of the flaxseed.

Because Sandy is receiving so many positive effects from her other supplements, and because the benefits of soy don't outweigh the possible risk of soy supplementation, soy is not included in her diet or list of prescribed supplements.

Chapter Lesson-There are numerous dietary supplements that have been CLINICALLY PROVEN to help fight breast cancer in a number of ways. I've purposefully not included doses for most supplements because it's important to work with your naturopathic doctor to determine the best regimen for YOU. If you decide to use traditional therapies, supplements can make them more effective and produce fewer side effects. If you elect, as Sandy has, to rely mainly on a natural approach which focuses on health, the use of supplements can replace traditional therapies and may provide results which are equal if not better to the use of traditional medications without their side effects.

*Sandy's Thoughts: What can I say except that supplements form a very important part of my treatment regimen. All of these supplements have been selected based upon a lot of research to help reduce inflammation in my body, replace bad fats with good fats, boost my immune system, and reduce my levels of bad estrogen. While there are no guarantees, I believe the supplements used in my treatment will help me as much if not more than conventional medicines in keeping my cancer away and keeping me healthy. I would agree with Shawn that it is vitally important for you to work with a doctor skilled in the treatment of cancer using nutritional supplements.*

*Just because I'm taking something doesn't mean it would be best for you. As is true with drug therapy, supplement therapy must be individualized to each person's needs and each person's type of cancer. Find someone you can trust and work with that person to develop the best supplement regimen for yourself.*

# Chapter 14

## *Preventing Cancer*

*It's better to prevent cancer than treat it.*

While there are many ideas I've already presented in *Breast Choices for the Best Chances: Your Breasts, Your Life, and How You Can Win the Battle!* to help you fight cancer and likely reduce or prevent future cancers, I'm going to share information given by Dr. Mercola (www.mercola.com) and others that I've found particularly helpful. Since only about 10% of cancers are genetic (inherited) in origin, this means that most cancers are related to environmental influences, most of which we can control (and thereby reduce our risks of developing cancer.)

1.Normalize your Vitamin D levels. So many people are vitamin D deficient and it is felt that many chronic diseases are caused by low vitamin D levels (and maybe can be prevented and/or treated with vitamin D supplementation.)

2.Control your insulin levels by limiting your intake of processed foods and sugars/fructose as much as possible. High insulin levels, which can cause insulin resistance, contribute to many chronic diseases.

3.Get appropriate amounts of animal-based omega-3 anti-inflammatory fatty acids. The typical Western diet is high in omega-6 fatty acids which tend to promote inflammation and disease.

4.Exercise. One of the primary reasons exercise works is that it drives your insulin levels down, and controlling insulin levels is one of the best powerful ways to reduce your cancer risks. Exercise also reduces stress, and stress contributes to many diseases. Studies have shown that breast cancer patients who exercise moderately for three to five hours a week cut their odds of dying from cancer by about half, compared to sedentary patients. In fact, any amount of weekly exercise increases your odds of surviving breast cancer. This benefit remained constant in studies regardless of whether women were diagnosed early or after their cancer had spread. The benefit of physical activity was particularly apparent among women with hormone-responsive tumors.

5.Eat healthy natural, preferably organic fresh food, especially colored vegetables (especially cruciferous vegetables) and fruits. Diets high in (organic) fruits and vegetables tend to cause less inflammation than diets based predominantly on animal proteins.

6.Relax! It is estimated that 85 percent of disease is caused by emotions or affected by negative emotions and stress due to chronically elevated cortisol levels.

7.Maintain proper body weight. Obesity contributes to many health problems. Fat serves as an endocrine organ and produces extra "bad" estrogens.

8.Get enough sleep. Rest is important for maintaining health.

9.Reduce your exposure to environmental toxins including pesticides, household chemical cleaners, synthetic air fresheners, xenoestrogens (chemicals which act like estrogens and can stimulate breast cancer,) and air pollution. Some of these toxins have been linked to various cancers including breast cancer.

10. Reduce your use of cell phones and other wireless technologies; excessive exposure to electromagnetic frequencies may contribute to disease.

11. Boil, poach or steam your foods, rather than frying or charbroiling them. If you must "fry," try sautéing with healthy olive oil.

12. Take supplements to maintain health and prevent disease.

13. If you like to eat meat, try organic meats, grass-fed meats, and organic wild game. Organic meats do not contain estrogens and growth hormones commonly used in the beef and dairy industries (if you like milk products, go organic.) Grass fed animals have healthier omega-3:omega-6 ratios and are less "inflammatory."

14. Minimize sugar intake to reduce insulin levels and insulin spikes.

15. Don't use chemical sugar substitutes (artificial sweeteners) which are excitotoxins.

## Common Environmental Xenoestrogens

Alkylphenols-intermediate chemicals used in the manufacture of other chemicals

Atrazine-weedkiller

4-methylbenzylidene camphor (4-MBC)-sunscreen lotions

Butylated hydroxyanisole( BHA)-food preservative

Bisphenol A-monomer for polycarbonate plastic and epoxy resin; antioxidant in plasticizers

Erythrosine- FD&C Red No. 3 dye

Ethinylestradiol-oral birth control pill-released into the environment as a xenoestrogen

Parabens- lotions

Phthalates-plasticizer

*Sandy's Thoughts: Chemotherapy doesn't cure cancer. Radiation therapy doesn't cure cancer. Surgery usually doesn't cure cancer (unless it's caught early.) While these modalities may help aid in the treatment of cancer (for those people who would truly benefit from them,) ultimately your immune system cures cancer and prevents more cancer. Unless you focus on health and improve your health with the many ideas Shawn and I have presented in Breast Choices for the Best Chances: Your Breasts, Your Life, and How You Can Win the Battle!, your immune system may not be able to cure you of your cancer. Lifestyle changes require work but ultimately lead to health. Whatever you do, you must focus on health and strengthening your immune system in order to have the best chance of surviving your cancer, preventing more cancer, and living a healthy, happy, and long life.*

# Chapter 15

# *Tests for The Woman With Breast Cancer*

*A few simple tests can increase your knowledge and open up a world of options.*

In order to get a diagnosis of breast cancer and properly stage the cancer, the typical woman has gone through numerous tests. However, there are some tests which I believe are VITALLY important in helping you beat your cancer and improve your odds, tests which your (conventional) doctor may or may not recommend to you. Here are 5 which Sandy and I believe are very helpful for the woman with breast cancer.

## Oncotype DX

The Oncotype DX test is performed after breast cancer surgery. The test examines 21 genes in YOUR tumor to determine a numerical value called your recurrence score. The recurrence score can tell you whether or not you have a low, intermediate, or high risk of your cancer returning in the future. It is recommended for women with estrogen receptor positive tumors.

The test has been validated (proven accurate) in pre- and postmenopausal women diagnosed with Stage I or Stage II invasive cancer with estrogen receptor positive tumors who have negative lymph nodes upon biopsy. The test can provide information to help you determine the best course of treatment: whether or not chemotherapy and/or tamoxifen therapy are appropriate. It also tries to give some idea of the likelihood of cancer returning in the future. In general, the recurrence score is usually associated with tumor size and even more so with tumor grade (smaller tumors and low grade aggressive tumors tend to have low recurrence scores.) Combining recurrence score, tumor grade, and tumor size provides better risk classification than any one of these factors alone.

Women with a low recurrence score have a low risk of cancer recurrence, so chemotherapy is unlikely to be of substantial benefit to them. Women with a high recurrence score have a high risk of cancer recurrence, so chemotherapy is likely to be of substantial benefit to them.
A woman with an intermediate score may or may not benefit from chemotherapy; and a discussion with her oncologist and naturopathic doctor is necessary to help the woman make the best decision regarding chemotherapy.

Based upon Sandy's low recurrence score of 15, she decided against chemotherapy.

Since the test is also validated for women who take tamoxifen, we used her recurrence score as a guideline to try to get some sort of grasp of the likelihood of a recurrence of Sandy's cancer if she decided against the use of tamoxifen. Based upon studies comparing the recurrence score's ability to predict recurrence in women treated with tamoxifen (at 10 years following diagnosis, the risks for breast cancer death in ER-positive, tamoxifen-treated patients with low recurrence score were 2.8%) versus women not treated with tamoxifen (at 10 years, the risks for breast cancer death in ER-positive patients not treated with tamoxifen were 6.2%,)

Based upon these statistics, Sandy also made the

decision not to use tamoxifen.


## Vitamin D (25-OH Vitamin D)

Most people suffer from vitamin D deficiency and should receive supplemental vitamin D to maintain health. This is especially critical for people with cancer as decreased levels of vitamin D are associated with increased cancer risk. The 25-hydroxy vitamin D test is the most accurate way to measure how much vitamin D is in your body. Minimum levels are 35 ng/ml. For health, many naturopathic doctors recommend levels at least 50 ng/ml. For patients with cancer, a target of at least 60-80 ng/ml and preferably 80-100 ng/ml is recommended.

Total serum 25(OH)D is the total amount of vitamin D (Vitamin D2 and the biologically active D3) in your blood. Since vitamin D2 is not naturally present in the human body, if you do not use supplements that contains vitamin D2 your results will only show vitamin D3, the form typically present in supplements and which you get from sun exposure.

Sandy's current total vitamin D level is 80 ng/ml, which is within the target goal of 80-100 ng/dl.

Note:If you have your vitamin D level tested at a conventional doctor's office, it is not unusual for the doctor's office to call back and tell you your result is "normal." Do not accept this as a definitive answer. To most conventional doctors, a "normal" vitamin D level is at least 35 ng/ml. For the cancer patient, you must strive to get your level closer to the 80-100 ng/ml range. For people who want to reduce their risks of any cancers, shoot for at least a result of 50-60 ng/ml.

## C-Reactive Protein (CRP)

C-reactive protein (CRP) and acute phase serum amyloid A proteins (A-SAA) are nonspecific proteins produced by the liver and secreted into the blood in response to inflammation in the body (technically in response to cytokine chemicals interleukin-1, interleukin-6 and tumor necrosis factor.) CRP can elevate in response to inflammation associated with many diseases including heart disease, coronary artery disease, inflammatory bowel disease, arthritis, pelvic inflammatory disease, lupus, severe infection, and cancers.

Results of the CRP test to determine the presence of inflammatory disease (as well as the risk of developing a disease, especially heart disease,) are between 0- 3.0 mg/dL.

Risk is assessed as follows:

Low (risk)-CRP of 1.0 milligrams/deciliter (mg/dL) or less.

Average (risk)-CRP between 1.0 and 3.0 mg/dL.

High (risk)-CRP greater than 3.0 mg/dL.

A CRP level greater than 10 mg/dL is a sign of serious inflammation or infection.

A study published online March 16, 2009 in the *Journal of Clinical Oncology* showed that high levels of C-reactive protein may be associated with the risk of developing cancer and with earlier cancer death. People with high blood levels of CRP (greater than 3 mg/L) have a 30% greater risk of developing any cancer later in life, and were associated with the risk of developing lung and possibly colorectal cancers, compared with people with low CRP levels. Researchers also found that among people with cancer, those with high CRP levels prior to their diagnosis were 80% more likely to die sooner than people with cancer who did not have elevated CRP. The researchers stated it is unclear whether CRP is a marker of occult (hidden) cancers or whether chronic inflammation, characterized by high CRP levels, promotes cancer growth. High CRP levels were associated with lung and possibly colorectal cancer risk, but did not significantly raise breast cancer risk. However, for women with breast cancer, elevated levels of CRP (and A-SAA) were found to be associated with reduced overall survival, no matter what the patient's age, tumor stage, race or body mass index. Researchers noted that in the long-term, elevated levels of inflammatory markers predict a woman's chances of surviving after breast cancer diagnosis. Breast cancer patients who had SAA blood levels in the highest third of the group were three times more likely to die from their disease in the following seven years, compared to patients with the lowest-third amount. Correspondingly, women in the highest third of CRP levels had a two-fold increased risk of death. Cancer survivors with chronic inflammation may have higher risk of recurrence, resulting from the effects on cell growth of inflammatory processes, or the presence of cancer cells that induce inflammation.

CRP levels (and inflammation in the body) can be reduced through supplementation with fish (or krill) oil, antioxidants, and improved diet.

Sandy's CRP level is 0.77 mg/L.

Omega Fatty Acid Profile (Omega 6/Omega 3)

This test measures your amount of omega-3 fatty acids and omega-6 fatty acids, and compares the ratio of omega-6/omega-3. People have evolved on a diet with a ratio of omega-6 to omega-3 essential fatty acids (EFA) of approximately 1, whereas the typical

Western/American diets have a much higher ratio around 15/1-17/1. The typical Western diet is deficient in omega-3 fatty acids and has excessive amounts of omega-6 fatty acids compared with the diet (the Mediterranean diet) on which we evolved and upon which our gene pool was established.

Excessive amounts of omega-6 fatty acids (PUFA) and a very high omega-6/omega-3 ratio promote inflammation and cell damage which results in many diseases, including cardiovascular disease, cancer, and inflammatory and autoimmune diseases. Conversely, increased levels of omega-3 fatty acids (a low omega-6/omega-3 ratio) exert suppressive (anti-inflammatory) effects.

In general, ratios of omega-6 fatty acids/omega-3 fatty acids should be 2/1-5/1. A lower omega-6/omega-3 ratio in women with breast cancer is associated with decreased risk of recurrence and death.

There is no "correct" ratio that has yet been established, and some studies indicate that the optimal ratio may vary with the disease under consideration. This is consistent with the fact that chronic diseases are the result of many genes and many factors. Therefore, it is quite possible that the ideal treatment dose of omega-3 fatty acids will depend on the degree of severity of disease resulting from the genetic predisposition.

At the American Association for Cancer Research (AACR) Meeting (April 2010,) it was reported that a low dietary omega-6 to omega-3 fatty acid ratio reduces breast density in an animal model. Mammographic density was used as a surrogate marker for breast cancer risk in the study (women with dense breasts have a higher incidence of breast cancer.) Although consumption of omega-3 fatty acids has been reported to reduce risk of breast cancer, the optimal omega-

6/omega-3 ratio has not been established. Both omega-6 and omega-3 fatty acids are essential for normal development and biological functioning.

A high omega-6 diet did not cause any increase in mammary gland density in the rats so treated. However, density was found to be significantly reduced in the low omega-6 to omega-3 ratio group; reduced breast density is associated with reduced levels of breast cancer.

At the same meeting, a study was designed to investigate the anticancer effect of two important omega-3 fatty acids, docosahexaenoic acid (DHA) and eicosapentaenoic acid (EPA,) while focusing on the possible role of fatty acid-induced oxidative stress and apoptosis (cell death) as mechanisms for chemopreventive actions.

Using the MCF-7 line of human breast cancer cells and athymic nude mice, it was shown that docosahexaenoic acid and eicosapentaenoic acid both strongly reduced the viability and DNA synthesis of MCF-7 human breast cancer cells in culture, and that these fatty acids also promoted apoptosis. Accumulation of reactive oxygen species and activation of caspase 8 were found to be important to the induction of apoptotic cell death. The simultaneous presence of antioxidants or a selective inhibition or knockdown of caspase 8 each were found to greatly interfere with the cytotoxic effect of docosahexaenoic acid.

In the mouse experiments, it was found that feeding the animals with a 5% fish oil diet for six weeks significantly reduced the growth of implanted MCF-7 human breast cancer cells by inhibiting cancer cell proliferation and promotion of cell death. Analysis of fatty acid content in mouse plasma and tissues demonstrated that the 5% fish oil diet significantly increased docosahexaenoic acid and eicosapentaenoic acid levels in both normal (329%

increase) and cancerous mammary tissues (300%). The conclusion is that omega-3 fatty acids strongly inhibit human breast cancer proliferation through formation of reactive oxygen species and induction of apoptosis by caspase 8 activation.

Sandy's ratio of omega-6 fatty acids/omega-3 fatty acids is 1.99, which is excellent and shows very low levels of pro-inflammatory omega 6 fatty acids.


## Urinary 2 hydroxyestrone/16 hydroxyestrone (2-OH/16-OH)

The urinary (2-OH/16-OH) test detects the levels of and ratio of 2 types of estrogen, 2 hydroxyestrone and 16 hydroxyestrone. Briefly, there are 3 "types" of naturally occurring/naturally formed estrogen in a woman's body: estradiol (E2, the biologically active estrogen most often associated with breast cancer,) estrone (E1,) and estriol (E3.) In your body these are all produced from androgens (such as testosterone or androstenedione) through the actions of enzymes (such as aromatase.) Estrone is "weaker" and "safer" than estradiol, and in post-menopausal women more estrone is present than estradiol. "Estrogen" is produced primarily by developing follicles in the ovaries, the corpus luteum and the placenta; some estrogens are also produced in smaller amounts by other tissues such as liver, adrenal glands, and the breasts. These tissues are the primary sources of estrogen in post-menopausal women.

Estradiol is oxidized in the liver to estrone (E1) and then hydroxylated by various enzymes including P450 enzymes, 2-hydroxylase, and 16alpha.-hydroxylase, to mainly 2-hydroxyestrone (2-0HE1) and 16 alpha-hydroxyestrone (16a-OHE1,) respectively.

The biological properties of these two compounds are different: 16a-OHE1 is generally viewed as an estrogen agonist (has estrogenic effects) similar to estradiol, while 2-0HE1 is believed to have minimal biological activity (and is considered a "safer" estrogen.) Therefore it has been suggested that the 2/16a-OHE1 ratio may be a test of breast cancer risk (the lower the ratio the higher the potential risk of breast cancer, or put differently the more 16-OH estrone you have the higher your breast cancer risk.)

Note:This is a very simple explanation of estrogen metabolism and testing. Other types of estrogen for which you can be tested include "good" estrogens such as 2-hydroxyestradiol (2-OHE2), 2-methoxyestrone (2-OMeE1) and 4-methoxyestrone (4-OMeE1) all of which have anti-cancer effects, as well as "bad" estrogens such as 4-hydroxyestrone which may react negatively with damaged DNA and contribute to cancer formation.

2-OH/16-OH ratios less than 2.0 indicate increasing long-term risk for breast, cervical, and other estrogen sensitive cancers due to higher levels of the "bad" 16-OH estrogen.  There is no "target" goal or "ideal" number at this time for which you should shoot for on your test, only striving to get it to at least 2.0. Sandy's current level is 14.2, indicating a preponderance of "good" estrogen in her body. This is likely due to numerous supplements she is taking that help create a favorable estrogen profile, but especially her cruciferous vegetable supplement (which contains high levels of cancer fighting chemicals such as I3C and DIM) and freshly ground flax seed. We will continue to monitor her urinary levels of 2-OH/16-OH as she makes adjustments to her supplement regimen.

Chapter Lesson-Even if your doctor does not order these tests, find a way to get them done! Doing so can mean the difference between life and death for the woman with breast cancer. And if you don't have cancer, some of the tests, such as for Vitamin D levels, CRP, and fatty acid ratios can guide your use of supplements and improve your health (and maybe reduce your chances of ever developing cancer.)

*Sandy's Thoughts:I believe these tests are all valuable for the woman who wants to prevent cancer or who has breast cancer. Unfortunately, most conventional cancer doctors will not prescribe them. You must ask for these yourself. If you can't convince your doctor to order them, you can order them yourself through Life Extension Foundation. I use the results of these to let me know just how well my supplements are working and to allow me to adjust the dosages of the supplements as needed. Finally I want to mention one thing about the vitamin D test. The "normal" range for vitamin D testing is between 35-100 ng/ml, yet all the research shows that 35 is way too low, especially for people with cancer. Most naturopathic cancer doctors recommend that your level should be at least 50 to maintain health and closer to 80-100 ng/ml to help fight and prevent cancer. If your doctor's office calls and reports your vitamin D level as "normal," you MUST get the actual numerical value of your test in order to know if you are at a proper level, rather than just accepting that your level is "normal."*

# Chapter 16

# *Final Thoughts*

*"Supporting the Fighters, Admiring the Survivors, Honoring the Taken, and NEVER, NEVER giving up hope."*

Jane Iscaro, Breast Cancer Survivor and Patient Advocate

To summarize the lessons Sandy and I have shared with you in prior chapters:

While we don't always know the exact cause of each person's cancer, there is no question that we live in a more toxic world today than Sandy and I lived in as children. We are constantly exposed to microwaves; radio waves (think cell phones;) estrogen-mimicking compounds in our plastic containers; synthetic hormones in birth control pills (often taken by girls at younger and younger ages for a variety of "medical problems;") hormone replacement therapy (which contains hundreds of estrogenic compounds, most of which don't even occur in the human body, prepared from horse urine;) antibiotics, growth hormones, and estrogens in our food supply; high fructose corn syrup (which increases our sugar load and leads to insulin resistance, a common cause of cancer development and growth;) partially hydrogenated vegetable oils; contaminated water; and heavy metals. Common sense as well as scientific research shows the harm that comes about from repeated exposure to these compounds.

Our diets are horrible. We eat mainly processed foods loaded with chemicals to keep them fresh for months or years. We rarely eat organic foods. We eat much more meat (hormone and antibiotic laden) than fruits and vegetables. We eat fish that is caught in chemically contaminated waters or farmed (and raised in farm ponds containing chemicals and hormones.)

"Exercise" means, for far too many Americans, lifting a fork from a plate containing unhealthy foods up to our mouths to have yet another portion of processed food that we do not need and which contributes to inflammation our bodies.

Most Americans are overweight, despite all of the evidence showing that obesity leads to a whole host of diseases including cancers.

Few of us take daily nutritional supplements (fish oil or antioxidants) proven to counteract the bad pro-inflammatory things we encounter every day.

We over-vaccinate our children and our pets, making them more likely to develop chronic diseases such as cancers without adding positively to their health.

Most of us are vitamin D deficient, yet don't take vitamin D supplements or get exposure to direct sunshine, both of which have been proven to counter depression, decreased libido, osteoporosis, and poorly functioning immune systems.

Most of us, especially our children who are forced to do hours of unnecessary homework, rarely get more than 4-6 hours of sleep per night.

We rarely have meaningful sex with our married partners, even though regular sexual encounters are beneficial for our emotional, spiritual, and physical health.

Stress is rampant: so much to do, so little time to rest/pray/have fun/build relationships/exercise/make love/enjoy life. Too much emotional garbage elevates our insulin and cortisol levels which predispose us to many chronic diseases, including cancer.

We over-medicate ourselves, both with prescription medications (most of which are not needed,) tobacco, illegal drugs, or alcohol.

When we become ill, our conventionally-trained doctors give us more conventional drugs, (most of which we do not need and which create new diseases or side effects which require more drugs to control,) rather than using diet, mind-body medicine, exercise, nutritional supplements, and other natural therapies such as chiropractic care or homeopathy that allow us to heal our own problems.

Some who read this book (and my other books) may incorrectly conclude that I am against conventional medicine and conventional therapies in the treatment of cancer. Nothing could be further from the truth. I am IN FAVOR of therapies that are necessary for and offer the most benefit to help people and pets recover from their diseases, whether they are conventional or natural. I AM AGAINST any therapy which does not offer significant help for the patient, and I am against a "one treatment is right for everyone" approach.

There is no "right" therapy for treating your cancer. The "right" therapy is the one YOU choose based upon all of the available information at your disposal. Whatever YOU choose, do not look back. YOUR choice is YOUR choice. Sandy has made numerous choices about her health. Whatever happens in the future, there are no regrets.

Hippocrates stated "Let food be your medicine," and "Above all do no harm." How many doctors follow these wise words of wisdom?

Just one day before losing her battle to cancer, Elizabeth Edwards wrote the following message on her Facebook page.

"You all know that I have been sustained throughout my life by three saving graces: my family, my friends, and a faith in the power of resilience and hope," she wrote. "These graces have carried me through difficult times and they have brought more joy to the good times than I ever could have imagined."

"The days of our lives, for all of us, are numbered. We know that. And, yes, there are certainly times when we aren't able to muster as much strength and patience as we would like. It's called being human."

"But I have found that in the simple act of living with hope, and in the daily effort to have a positive impact in the world, the days I do have are made all the more meaningful and precious. And for that I am grateful."

Here are some closing thoughts Sandy and I wish to share with you. I wish I could claim credit for them but I cannot. These thoughts are adapted from Kate Nowak's poem "May You Be Blessed":

May you be blessed with all things good.

May your joys, like the stars at night, be too numerous to count.

May your victories be more abundant than all the grains

of sand on all the beaches on all the oceans in all the world.

May lack and struggle only serve to make you stronger.

And may beauty, order and abundance be your constant companions.
May every pathway you choose lead to that which is pure and good and lovely.

May every doubt and fear be replaced by a deep, abiding trust as you observe
evidence of God all around you.

And where there is only darkness and the storms of life are closing in, may
the light of God illuminate your world.

May you always be aware that you are loved beyond measure and may you be
willing to strive to love unconditionally in return.

May you always feel protected and cradled in the arms of God like the cherished child you are.

And when you are tempted to judge, may you be reminded that God does not
want this for us, and that you are accountable for every word you utter.

And when you are tempted to hold back may you remember that love flows best
when it flows freely, and that it is in loving that we receive the greatest
gift.

May you always have music and laughter and may a rainbow follow every storm.

May gladness wash away every disappointment.

May joy dissolve every sorrow and may love ease every pain.

May every wound bring wisdom and may every trial bring triumph.

And with each passing day may you live more abundantly than the day before.

May you be blessed and may others be blessed by you.


This is my heartfelt prayer for you: May you be blessed.


*"When you're weak, I'll be strong / When you let go, I'll hold on / When you need to cry, I swear that I'll be there to dry your eyes / When you feel lost and scared to death, like you can't take one more breath / Just take my hand, together we can do this / I'm gonna love you through it,"*

From *"I'm Gonna Love You Through It"*

Martina McBride


And remember, above all else, it is...*Your Breasts and Your Life, and You Can Win the Battle!*

# What Others Are Saying About *Breast Choices for the Best Chances: Your Breasts, Your Life, and How You Can Win the Battle!*

*"Breast Choices for the Best Chances: Your Breasts, Your Life, and How You Can Win the Battle!* is a masterpiece! It is the best advice I have ever seen for women dealing with breast cancer, and the information is presented in very logical, easy-to- read and understandable language, and strongly backed by research.

Sandy and Shawn Messonnier have written not only a personal account of her experiences with a disease most women fear beyond imagination, but they have produced one of the best books on the issue I have ever seen. Their work is not only well written, easy to understand and written with a beautiful prose, but the information is presented logically throughout the entire book and backed by some of the best science available. I was especially pleased with the information in the chapter on statistics and the mammography controversy. Every chapter takes women through clear explanations of each step in their travels through this mysterious and often frightening world and gives them confidence and hope. I am also pleased that Sandy openly shares her faith and the importance of faith in dealing with this disease—even when the results are not as one hoped. Every woman should carefully read this wonderful work from Sandy's heart."

Russell L. Blaylock, M.D.
Author: Natural Strategies for Cancer Patients
www.blaylockwellnesscenter.com
www.russellblaylockmd.com

"As someone who has been in the trenches treating cancer patients for the past 24 years, I can recommend Dr. Messonnier's wonderful new book, *Breast Choices for the Best Chances:Your Breasts, Your Life, and How You Can Win the Battle!* about breast cancer without reservation.  He has taken up a most difficult challenge, chronicling his wife's fight with the disease, while at the same time weaving in thoroughly researched information from both conventional and more alternative sources.

The book combines the best of all possible worlds, a moving personal story of a patient dealing with a potentially deadly diagnosis, combined with high scholarship and useful practical advice

I have followed Dr. Messonnier's pioneering work with animals for years, and have long appreciated his sound scholarship and creative approach to disease.  In *Breast Choices for the Best Chances:Your Breasts, Your Life, and How You Can Win the Battle!,* his many years of training and study shine through.

As I read the book, I so appreciated his determination to provide the reader with the latest concepts about breast cancer, without dismissing any approach, whether traditional or not.  Using his wife's situation as a starting point he discusses the rationale and statistics for standard approaches to breast cancer such as chemotherapy and hormonal blockade. He then provides a most detailed analysis of alternative and nutritional therapies ranging from anti-oxidants and herbs to indole-3-carbinol.  His documentation is sound, and his analysis of breast cancer pathology is particularly insightful, pointing out as he does so clearly the confusion in the field that often leads to bad decisions and unnecessary aggressive treatment.

Dr. Messonnier is to be commended for providing such a thoughtful rendering of his family situation, as he and his wife sought to find the best approach to her condition.

And he has done us all a great favor, by giving us such a much-needed analysis of breast cancer, its treatment possibilities, and showing us that even in the darkest of times, solutions can be certainly found."

Nick Gonzalez, M.D.

http://www.dr-gonzalez.com/index.htm

*"Breast Choices for the Best Chances:Your Breasts, Your Life, and How You Can Win the Battle!* is a valuable book to read for anyone touched by the nightmare known as cancer. It is very important for people (and their families) who have been given this diagnosis, to feel that they can navigate through the treacherous waters of modern oncology, and to find a treatment program that works for them. It is important for them to know that they do not have to follow the "slash, burn and poison" approach of modern medicine. Bravo to Shawn for taking the time, energy and effort to produce such a work!


Robert A. Eslinger, D.O., H.M.D.
Medical Director
Reno Integrative Medical Center
Reno, NV

"*Breast Choices for the Best Chances* is a valuable resource for anyone concerned about breast cancer. Dr. Messonnier provides a good overview of the risk factors and conventional therapies for breast cancer, as well as his areas of special expertise, namely, the nutritional approaches to preventing cancer and supporting conventional treatment.

In particular, Dr. Messonnier's discussion of dietary fats -- especially omega-3 and omega-6 fatty acids – illuminates the increasingly well-documented roles that inflammation and cell signaling play in cancer's genesis. I recommend *Breast Choices for the Best Chances* to all women and their families."

Craig Weatherby

Editor of "Vital Choices" health letter and co-author (with Leonid Gordin, M.D.) of *The Arthritis Bible* (Healing Arts Press 1999)

Vital Choice Wild Seafood & Organics

www.vitalchoice.com

"Dr. Messonnier is a naturopathic/holistic veterinarian, who wrote this book to help women make their own informed choices regarding their own healthcare, as well as to help those charities he felt were most in need of his financial support. It is the story of his wife Sandy's successful fight with breast cancer, as well as a sharing of the results of all of the research he found in his efforts to help her with this battle. He does an excellent job of explaining what tests are most helpful in obtaining the knowledge a woman needs to make an informed decision regarding her treatment. He also provides a summary of the research results currently available in order to know how to interpret those tests and to fully understand what stage one's cancer is in. In addition, he offers an explanation of the many supplements one can take to minimize one's risks and to serve as an adjunct to conventional therapies. Although he believes that an integrative approach of conventional and alternative treatments is best, he does a great job of presenting the information so that each woman can make her own decisions about what is the most optimal approach for her.

*Breast Choices for the Best Chances: Your Breasts, Your Life, and How You Can Win the Battle!* is an excellent guideline for all women to aid them in the prevention and/or treatment of breast cancer. It is also an excellent resource for those serving in a supportive role, such as a husband or parent to a woman with breast cancer. I learned a great deal of valuable information while reading this book. I feel better informed and more knowledgeable on ways to stay healthy and what to do should I ever be confronted with this horrible illness. Although Dr. Messonnier found that not much progress has been made in the war on cancer, he feels that the world of integrative oncology does offer a lot of hope for the cancer patient. Of course, knowledge is power, and those wishing to prevent cancer or those diagnosed with cancer will find this book a must read.

As Dr. Messonnier says, given that "Cancer therapy is very much an individual and personal decision", it is important for people to have all of the information available in order to make the best decision possible for their particular situation and condition. He does a wonderful job of educating current and future cancer patients about all of their options. I feel that many people will benefit from the knowledge Dr. Messonnier gained on this journey with his wife."

Felicia Weiss, Ph.D.
Holistic Networker

"I love that *Breast Choices for the Best Chances: Your Breasts, Your Life, and How You Can Win the Battle!* is written from the perspective of a breast cancer survivor and her loving, caring husband. It is a great book that talks about alternatives other than the typical modern day medical perspective you might get from your oncologist and looks into things holistically, focusing on health and not disease.

When it comes to breast cancer people are hearing more about natural healing; this book also backs up recommendations with the proven facts from studies done on these alternative natural healing methods.

 I LOVE that the door is always open for more holistic ways of fighting disease and I hope one day it will be covered under health insurance for people and pets.

I have a small group of friends that are fighting for their lives and I have already lost a few from this disease. Every year I lose someone I have met to breast cancer. The information in *Breast Choices for the Best Chances: Your Breasts, Your Life, and How You Can Win the Battle!* will go a long way to saving lives that shouldn't be lost to this horrible disease.

Let's NEVER forget we need a cure and I want to see it in MY life time. NEVER give up HOPE for that to happen. With all the knowledge that is out there the CURE is around the corner and with the information in this book IT CAN HAPPEN.

Jane Iscaro
Breast cancer survivor and patient advocate

"Dr. Shawn Messonnier has hit a home run with this fabulous book about breast cancer. *Breast Choices for the Best Chances: Your Breasts, Your Life, and How You Can Win the Battle!* is powerful and informative. More importantly it provides a detailed road map for anyone dealing with breast cancer.  But the real star of this book is Shawn's wife Sandy, a courageous woman of God who met her own breast cancer head on.  She is proof positive that with the proper tools, information and support, breast cancer can be conquered. After reading this book it's clear that Shawn married UP!!! This book is a must read. Read it and prepared to be blessed."

David Timothy, a.k.a. The SoupMan
Executive Director---SoupMobile Inc
Author of *Is God On Vacation?* and *God is NOT on Vacation!*
Dallas, Texas
www.soupmobile.org

*"Breast Choices for the Best Chances:Your Breasts, Your Life, and How You Can Win the Battle!* is a moving account of the health and healing journey of Sandy Messonnier and her husband, Holistic Veterinarian, Dr. Shawn Messonnier. The book takes us through the myriad of issues they faced after her diagnosis of breast cancer. This moving personal account of their experience is interwoven with Dr. Messonnier's analysis of relevant research and statistics and Sandy's personal thoughts on the issues. From understanding basics about cancer, early diagnosis, surgical , hormonal, radiation, and chemotherapy decisions to the importance of loving relationships, a spiritual life, healthy diet and lifestyle, the book discusses the helpful information on all these areas. There is candid discussion of the risks and benefits of available conventional treatment options. The extensive supplemental support items they chose to add to Sandy's regimen are discussed though specific doses are not included, as Dr. Messonnier explains that supplemental decisions should involve individuals and their own health care providers.

I appreciate the extent of the medical research review and the plain spoken analysis of the many issues a woman newly diagnosed with breast cancer will have to contend with. I gained insight about the information used by the Messonniers in order to arrive at many of their decisions. With every breast cancer diagnosis there is an enormous amount of information to sort through to make informed decisions at every step of the journey. This beautiful account will hopefully help others facing similar concerns."

Anne Coleman, MD

*"Breast Choices for the Best Chances:Your Breasts, Your Life, and How You Can Win the Battle!* is a great combination of natural and conventional treatment options. Presenting both natural and conventional treatments empowers women to make informed decisions when it comes to their health.

*Breast Choices for the Best Chances:Your Breasts, Your Life, and How You Can Win the Battle!* is a MUST-HAVE book to help guide women who are experiencing breast cancer to find the solution that is right for them."

Andrea Donsky
Co-Founder, NaturallySavvy.com
Twitter.com/NaturallySavvy
Facebook.Com/NaturallySavvy

"I met Dr. Shawn Messonnier almost two years ago. I have a great deal of respect for him as a veterinarian, a husband and a father. In reading this book I learned that there are so many choices for women who are diagnosed with breast cancer. Cancer is a word that no one wants to hear. I feel this book is a must read for every women, whether you have had breast cancer or not. It is extremely important for women to know the options that are available to them in helping to prevent and treat breast cancer.

I think having the medical information in *Breast Choices for the Best Chances:Your Breasts, Your Life, and How You Can Win the Battle!* is a great idea. Reading "Sandy's thoughts" was very inspirational. We constantly hear about cancer from the medical professionals but rarely from the patient. The way Sandy talks about all the factors involved in her decision process was amazing. Cancer is different for everyone and the decisions on treatment should be evaluated carefully and on an individualized basis.

Thank you Sandy and Dr. Shawn for writing this book!!!!"

Mona Hall
Ron's Organic Dynamics

"Thank you Dr. Shawn, and your courageous wife Sandy, for sharing your story and cancer experience! It is critical for women (and men) to realize that surviving a life threatening illness such as cancer requires their active engagement in researching and understanding their treatment options. Your message will likely save the lives of many women who realize that they are entitled to a treatment plan that addresses their individual needs. Every day women lose their cancer battle because they were so overwhelmed by the diagnosis, that they accepted the "standard of care" without question. *Breast Choices for the Best Chances:Your Breasts, Your Life, and How You Can Win the Battle!* will empower women to truly understand their options for "customized care" with a road map to their own "breast choices" for survival."

Julie Joyce
Executive Producer & Host of Cancer Free Radio

"I learned a great deal from *Breast Choices for the Best Chances:Your Breasts, Your Life, and How You Can Win the Battle!* I believe that it offers a very interesting perspective and is very thought provoking. I do believe that it will empower women to explore other means of treating their breast cancer. I also believe that it will empower women to question and challenge their physicians to be sure that their treatment recommendations are truly personalized for their individual case. I believe that it can be very easy for practitioners to treat women with their standard protocol and possibly forget to consider what is truly best for that individual's treatment.

I really loved the personal feelings that you Shawn and Sandy shared throughout *Breast Choices for the Best Chances:Your Breasts, Your Life, and How You Can Win the Battle!* I think that when a person goes through a cancer diagnosis, it helps to see that others have had similar feelings. I also think that your book shows the importance of every patient having an advocate to help them sort through the information they are given and to help them to make "informed" rather than "scared" decisions. And you truly show the benefit of having an advocate who has medical knowledge who can really decipher the information they are given."


Lisa Venincasa, R.N.

"*Breast Choices for the Best Chances:Your Breasts, Your Life, and How You Can Win the Battle!* is an inspiring story of strength under the ultimate challenge. Sandy's courage is an inspiration that can help other women overcome fear and confusion to make the best choices for their own health. Bravo!"

Tracie Hotchner

Author, *The Dog Bible, The Cat Bible*, and *Pregnancy & Childbirth*

As a professional journalist, I tend to look at all new things with a skeptical eye. I did this as I read Dr. Messonnier's book, "*Breast Choices for the Best Chances:Your Breasts, Your Life, and How You Can Win the Battle!* But I must say that I am honestly impressed. He has done great research and bases his thoughts on facts, not just opinions. I wish this book had been around when my mother was going through her years of cancer and treatment. This is truly a book that could be beneficial to practically everyone. It contains useful information on nutrition and supplements, and how they can be used to help reduce the odds of cancer ever taking place. Cancer can be a terrifying proposition, but Dr. Messonnier has a way of saying, "OK, it's cancer. We still have control of our bodies. Now, here are our options." Well done.

Sam Moore, former News Director WAPT-TV, Jackson MS

# Addendum-DCIS

DCIS, short for ductal carcinoma in situ, is diagnosed with greater frequency since mammography has become routine for most women. DCIS is not a tumor and cannot typically be felt by the woman or doctor. Rather, it is a diagnosis that is made by imaging (mammography, MRI, etc.) The widespread use of screening mammography has led to numerous diagnoses of DCIS. It is unlikely that the frequency of DCIS has risen (although that is possible,) but rather the diagnosis has risen due to many more women receiving mammograms. As a result, it is diagnosed more frequently now that mammography has become commonplace, and DCIS is diagnosed more frequently and treated more aggressively in the USA than in other countries.

While the incidence of DCIS has continued to rise in younger, premenopausal women (possibly due to normal hormonal influence, increased exposure to environmental hormones, increased use of hormonal birth control, etc.,) the incidence has decreased in postmenopausal women since standard "hormone therapy" is no longer used for most women.

Note:When you see statistics mentioning how fewer women are dying from breast cancer, that is because DCIS is being included in the cancer diagnostic database. Since most women with DCIS are in no danger of dying, it makes sense that including them among women with more aggressive (and more likely fatal) breast cancer would artificially lower the mortality rate.

This is another way that cancer statistics can be skewered to show a favorable response.

Many doctors question whether or not DCIS should be considered a "cancer," a "precancerous lesion," an "intermediate step" between normal breast tissue and early invasive carcinoma, or a "suspicious radiographic anomaly" that may or may not ever cause a problem.

In fact, the reported incidence of death from breast cancer in patients diagnosed with DCIS is less than 2%. This brings up the question of how a woman diagnosed with only DCIS through routine mammography should be treated, or whether or not treatment is even needed.

It is beyond the scope of this book to delve too deeply into this topic, but the following points will be helpful in guiding your decision if you are ever diagnosed with DCIS.

1. In most cases, DCIS is nonaggressive and treatment can also be nonaggressive. Statistically, regardless of conventional treatment, most cases of DCIS (the non-comedo type which is essentially nonaggressive) have a low mortality rate. Many doctors think of DCIS in women, especially older women, similar to early nonaggressive prostate cancer that, especially if diagnosed in men over the age of 70, may never develop into an aggressive cancer.

2. A biopsy of the area can help determine if the DCIS is anything to be worried about. In most instances, the pathology shows a relatively benign lesion that may not warrant further conventional therapy, especially if the biopsy shows no remaining DCIS or other abnormalities.

3.For localized lesions, while some doctors recommend aggressive therapy with radiation and/or tamoxifen, these may not be needed in cases of benign pathology reports. More aggressive lesions (comedo formation) may prompt the oncologist to more aggressively recommend these conventional therapies, but studies have not shown a difference in survival.

This is obviously an area that requires accurate information and thought on the part of the woman diagnosed with DCIS. If my daughter were to be diagnosed with DCIS, I would recommend the following after explaining to her that the natural history of most cases of DCIS is unknown which results in a dilemma in not being able to distinguish which lesions will be associated with a subsequent invasive cancer:

1.Consider a biopsy to determine if it is the rare slightly more aggressive form or the more common benign form. Only do the biopsy after starting supplements such as modified citrus pectin and cimetidine to reduce the chance of any "cancerous" cells from spreading during the biopsy.

2.Watching and waiting can be an acceptable alternative to surgery IF you will also start an aggressive cancer fighting supplement protocol, focusing especially on vitamin D, fish oil, and an anti-estrogen cruciferous vegetable supplement (of course my daughter and your daughter should already be taking some of these supplements to maximize health and prevent cancer; doing so makes it less likely that our daughters will ever develop DCIS or breast cancer.)

3.Have another test (mammogram, MRI, etc.) in 3-6 months following the supplement regimen (especially if the lesion was not biopsied) to determine if the natural approach cured the DCIS (which is likely to happen.)

Finally, I would share the following information with her to help guide her choice.

"Mortality from breast cancer is low among women diagnosed with DCIS regardless of the type of treatment women undergo. Only 1.0%–2.6% of women diagnosed with DCIS will die of invasive breast cancer within 8–10 years of diagnosis. Whether the low risk of death from breast cancer is because of very effective treatments or the fact that the majority of DCIS are relatively benign, or both, are unclear. *There are no data that demonstrate detection of DCIS by mammography averts breast cancer deaths. Thus, screening mammography may be benefiting some women whose DCIS would be associated with subsequent invasive cancer, whereas it is potentially harming other women whose DCIS would never be associated with subsequent invasive cancer, who for lack of good prognostic indicators, are almost always treated with surgery and adjuvant therapies.*"

Epidemiology of Ductal Carcinoma In Situ, Karla Kerlikowske, JCNI Monographs, Volume 2010, Issue 41, pages 139-141.

# About Shawn and Sandy Messonnier

Shawn Messonnier, DVM, is the author of numerous books on natural pet care including the award-winning *The Natural Health Bible for Dogs & Cats*. He is also the host of the award-winning radio show on Martha Stewart Living Radio on Sirius/XM 110, *Dr. Shawn-The Natural Vet*. Utilizing a holistic approach in his practice, Paws & Claws Animal Hospital, he teaches pet owners how to keep their pets healthy and reduce and treat illness using natural therapies.

Sandy Messonnier is a housewife and mother and has a degree in marketing. She believes strongly in living life to the fullest and staying healthy. She is committed to sharing her story and her belief in the benefits of exercise, prayer, relaxation, good diet, and the proper use of nutritional supplements as a foundation for health.

# Afterword

*"Survival is the ultimate test to determine if a therapy is working."*

Dr. Nicholas Gonzalez

*"If only I had listened to the voice inside."*

Kathy, Breast Cancer Victim

Sandy and I hope this book has been a source of inspiration and information for you. If you are ever diagnosed with cancer, we know how terrifying that can be for you. We believe the information in " *Breast Choices for the Best Chances: Your Breasts, Your Life, and How You Can Win the Battle!* will help give you unbiased factual information that lets you make the best decision for yourself.

Whatever you do, you must move past fear, as fear encourages irrational decisions.

It's important to have a strong support group of friends and family members. Sandy found comfort in the fact that I was always there for her and that our daughter Erica did not "freak out" and become uncomfortable around her following Sandy's diagnosis.

Sandy's friends from her church group were also very supportive. Friends and family may not know how to act around you once they hear the diagnosis of "cancer" as this diagnosis often causes fear in them and evokes thoughts of pain, misery, and certain death. Obviously most women who are diagnosed with early stage invasive breast cancer will live normal lives once they choose the proper therapies for themselves. You may need to have open and frank discussions with your friends and family members so they know what to expect as well as how to act around you (hint-they need to act normal around you!)

Sandy found that many people in her group called to check on her quite a bit following her initial diagnosis and treatment, but once they knew she was okay the volume of calls decreased. This is normal and to be expected. It does not mean that your friends no longer care about you, only that they have returned to their normal behavior once they know you do not need the extra attention.

If you find that your cancer is more advanced or recurs, keep an open mind to every and any possible therapy, including chemotherapy trials of new medications or new treatment regimens. Also stay open to the possibility of unusual naturopathic treatments such as antineoplaston therapy (offered by Dr. Stanislaw Burzynski, http://www.burzynskiclinic.com, and pancreatic enzyme therapy (offered by Dr. Nick Gonzalez, http://www.dr-gonzalez.com/index.htm.)

Sandy has found a lot of comfort with friends and family, exercise, relaxation, and prayer. Find what works best for you and realize you are not alone on your journey. And feel free to contact us through my website, www.petcarenaturally.com.

www.ingramcontent.com/pod-product-compliance
Lightning Source LLC
Chambersburg PA
CBHW050124280326
41933CB00010B/1242